Overcoming IBS

This book is dedicated to our parents

OVERCOMING IBS

Practical Help in Coping with Irritable Bowel Syndrome

Christine P. Dancey
and Susan Backhouse

Robinson Publishing
LONDON

Robinson Publishing
7, Kensington Church Court
London W8 4SP

First published by Robinson Publishing 1993

A copy of the British Library Cataloguing in Publication
Data for this title is available from the British Library.

ISBN 1-85487-175-7

Typeset by Hewer Text Composition Services, Edinburgh
Printed in Great Britain by the Guernsey Press Ltd.

Contents

Acknowledgements

We would like to thank: Professor Nick Read for support throughout the time the Network has been in existence, and for reading the manuscript and making important suggestions and additions for clarification; Michael Johnstone for reading the manuscript and making helpful suggestions; Carol Backhouse for reading through parts of the manuscript and offering the benefit of her astute eye; Anne Woolett and Harriette Marshall of the University of East London for reading through parts of the manuscript; Kathy Armes for her enthusiastic response to the chapters she read; Carole Scanlon for information on relaxation techniques; Lynn Hardcastle for sharing her nutritional expertise; Dr Chris Mallinson and Professor Wingate for support, encouragement, and time; Ann Stapleton in the Psychology office of the University of London for help in preparing the manuscript for printing; and all the members of the IBS Network who contributed to the book by talking and writing about their IBS.

Sue would particularly like to thank Philip, and also Kenneth Backhouse for the time to write this book, and Chris Backhouse for his interest and enthusiasm. Christine would like to thank Michael Davey, Jo Johnstone and Maureen O'Hara for support and encouragement during the writing of this book.

Foreword

This is a book written by sufferers for sufferers concerning a disease that tends to be disregarded by many of the medical profession as a somatic manifestation of a neurotic personality, a condition not worthy of their time and expertise. Nevertheless, irritable bowel syndrome (IBS) exerts an enormous strain on health care resources. It affects about a quarter of the population and functional gastrointestinal disorders, of which IBS is the most commonly diagnosed condition, are said to comprise over 50 per cent of all referrals – yet there is no real agreement on how to treat them.

Diseases like IBS are a casualty of the development of 'scientific medicine', the magic bullet approach. This consists of identifying the disease by means of tests and then administering a specific tablet to treat it. However, there is no specific test for IBS: blood levels, X-rays and even biopsies of the bowel are usually quite normal. None of the advances of drug therapy and diagnosis have really benefited the patient with IBS, and in adopting the magic bullet approach health workers may have lost touch with the traditional and more holistic approach to medicine. I suspect that diseases like IBS were better managed in the past when doctors and their patients were more attuned to, and more accepting of, the relationship between the mind and the body. Yet IBS is being diagnosed more and more frequently.

So what is IBS? It should not be used as a convenient catch-all for all those gut diseases that are not characterized by inflammation, ulceration or cancer. In a major subset of patients, the gut appears to become sensitized to the presence of food, distension, the production of gas, the formation of chemicals – in fact, all the normal events that take place during the digestive process. This sensitization may be triggered by stress, a particular personality or a harrowing lifestyle, but it can also be induced by more visceral factors, such as a previous gastrointestinal infection, an operation on the pelvis such as a hysterectomy, or impaired absorption of bile acids from the intestine. It is demeaning to the patient to imply that IBS is exclusively a psychosomatic condition. I have heard it said that IBS patients find it difficult to express their anger. Just try asking them what they think about their doctors!

Susan Backhouse and Christine Dancey have written an original and powerful book that draws on the experience of the large number of IBS sufferers who, in their frustration with the medical profession, have joined the IBS Network. This is a self-help group which Christine and Susan have established as a forum for IBS sufferers to share their experiences, to express their frustrations and to find out for themselves what treatments work for them. In joining the IBS Network, the patients are sending out a clear signal to the medics: they are saying, 'Look, most of you are not able to offer us anything of any use. We are going to try to help ourselves to manage this condition.' The gauntlet has been cast down in front of the champions of the National Health Service to challenge their attitudes to IBS and perhaps all 'functional disease'. Perhaps they should recommend a more holistic approach that looks at the disease in relation to the person, his or her environment, diet and life experience. The problem, as always, is one of resource. How can doctors investigate fully the relationship between the person and his or her disease in a single five-minute interview? No wonder both doctors and patients become frustrated.

There must be another way of tackling such diseases. Perhaps doctors can work with self-help groups to enable patients to take responsibility for their condition by providing insights into the origin of symptoms, the linkage between life experiences and disease and the simple changes that might be attempted to alleviate the condition. Self-help groups are an important development, but they should not be an alternative to conventional medical management. Instead, doctors and self-help groups should learn to work together to tackle the enormous problem of functional disease.

What Susan Backhouse and Christine Dancey are proposing is nothing short of a quiet revolution in health care. Their message could be applied to all functional diseases and many organic illnesses. It is important that this revolution occurs with the support, and, dare I say, guidance of the professionals. After all, surely our goals are the same! I wish the book and the IBS Network every success.

N. W. Read,
Professor of Gastrointestinal
Physiology and Nutrition,
the University of Sheffield
Northern General Hospital.

Preface

This is the book that we wanted years ago. Why has it only just been written? In September 1990 the authors of this book were searching (independently) for an irritable bowel syndrome self-help group, a search which proved futile, but one which put us in contact with each other. It was clear that despite the fact that an estimated 15 per cent of people suffer from IBS,[1] there was no organization, no self-help or support groups, no newsletter, nothing catering for the needs of IBS sufferers – so we decided we would set up such an organization ourselves. This became known as the IBS Network. Our main aim was to help alleviate the isolation of people diagnosed as having IBS by providing a means of contact with fellow-sufferers. This is being achieved firstly by way of a newsletter, which has facilitated the setting up of self-help groups, and now through the medium of this book.

We both suffer from IBS; one of us has had it for 20 years. Once we had contacted others with IBS, we quickly realized that what people wanted most of all was to be able to read about the experiences of others with the same disorder. They needed to know that other people were suffering the same ordeals, and were coping with them. The very few books on IBS describe the symptoms and speculate on its causes, yet none of them describe what it is like from the sufferer's point of view. Consequently, although people can read about the tests they have undergone and what may have caused their IBS, they cannot read about how painful the tests were, the feelings the test gave rise to, and how, when each test was shown to be negative, they felt as if they were a fraud; IBS has never had the validity of a 'real' disease. They have not been able to read about the embarrassment that the loud noises in the digestive system can bring, the lack of control felt when rushing to the toilet numerous times a day, and so on. Sufferers had no way of knowing how common their feelings were.

Apparently IBS was first described in 1820 by a gastroenterologist called Powell. Since then it has been called by various names, including spastic colon, spasmodic stricture of the colon, membranous enteritis and vegetative neurosis. IBS is a diagnosis of exclusion: once other, more serious diseases have been discounted (cancer of the bowel, Crohn's disease, colitis, coeliac diseases) IBS is diagnosed. It has no known causes, and no cure which is lastingly effective. Sufferers experience continuous or recurrent symptoms of abdominal pain, altered bowel habits, flatulence, early satiety, and bloating or a feeling of abdominal distension. Altered bowel habits may give rise to diarrhoea, constipation, or an alternation of both. Often there is straining or urgency, and a feeling of incomplete evacuation of the bowel.

IBS is responsible for a significant loss of work time, a large number of visits to doctors and frequent hospital admissions;[2] it accounts for 30 to 50 per cent of consultations to gastroenterologists.[3] However, despite the prevalence of this disorder, there is incomplete agreement on its definition and its status as a valid diagnostic entity and is not taken seriously by many doctors – something that can be very distressing if your life is being ruined by it.[4]

We sent out questionnaires to members of the IBS Network and their replies make a valuable contribution to this book. Respondents' names have all been changed. Our sample of IBS sufferers includes people of all ages and of both sexes. For some of them the symptoms were overwhelming; they were in a great deal of pain and found it hard to cope. Others had found their symptoms became more bearable as the years passed. Most of them expressed relief that they could finally talk about all their problems, without fear and embarrassment, knowing that other people understood. They found reassurance in the realization that there were others like them, and hope in the knowledge that some people manage to cope with their symptoms so well that IBS is a very small part of their lives.

As IBS cannot at present be cured and appears to have several causes, it is not a matter of simply going to your doctor to be diagnosed and successfully treated. The medical profession doesn't have any easy answers to this one. At the end of the day, if the treatments offered don't work, you may feel you are on your own.

We hope this book makes you realize you are not on your own. In it, many people suffering from IBS tell of their experiences, how they live with the condition and what they would like to see changed.

We ourselves are not medical practitioners. Our qualifications for writing *Overcoming IBS* are years of living with IBS and a strong desire to make other sufferers feel less helpless and alone.

Chapter 1

What Exactly Is IBS?

'My problems start with a pain, like a dull ache, in the lower abdomen, followed by the most incredible bloating ever seen in a non-pregnant woman, constipation, pain and a feeling of general malaise. This is eventually relieved by strong doses of Colpermin and laxatives.'

IBS is a digestive disorder characterized by unexplained abdominal pain, varying in intensity from mild to extremely severe, and altered bowel habits, which can include diarrhoea, constipation or an alternation of both, together with other symptoms discussed later in this chapter. The disorder can be fairly persistent, but is often characterized by times when the symptoms become very bad and remissions where the symptoms are much more manageable. IBS is a diagnosis of exclusion (although many doctors think it shouldn't be); once other, more serious, diseases have been excluded, and there are no signs of parasites or enzyme deficiency, the patient is given a diagnosis of IBS. IBS is termed a 'functional' disorder – which means that there is no actual disease which can account for the symptoms experienced.

IBS is probably a catch-all label for a variety of conditions with a variety of causes linked by a bowel disorder which doctors cannot identify or understand, nor treat effectively. In the past for instance, symptoms caused by lactose intolerance have come under the heading of IBS. Some researchers believe there are more IBS 'sub-groups' to be discovered and they are trying to develop tests to identify them. There is unlikely to be a miracle cure round the corner which will help all IBS sufferers.

1

How does IBS start?

Henry describes how his IBS started:

'I'm 30 now, and have had IBS to varying degrees for about seven years. I was never aware of having any bowel problems when a child. On a few occasions at school when I was 17 or 18 I remember feeling the need to go to the toilet during the day, but in general there was no urgency and I was able to last out until I got home. I had one period of a few months when I suffered severe flatulence which made me feel as if I needed a bowel movement, but wasn't actually able to do anything. I also became aware of occasionally needing to go to the toilet twice in the morning, or in the late afternoon or early evening, particularly if I was on holiday or had gone out for the day. A few years later, when I was in a job which I enjoyed, I found I only just had time to open the post before I needed to go to the toilet. It rapidly got worse, and I soon reached a situation where I was having to go three times in quick succession in the morning, and often suddenly at other times of the day as well, which quite worried me, as I thought it might be something serious. For a month or so the IBS was probably as bad as it ever has been since. I have never really had any clear idea of why IBS developed at this time.'

However, different people experience the start of their IBS in different ways – there is no common pattern of onset. Here some other sufferers describe how their IBS started.

'It all began a year ago while I had what I thought was indigestion. I took some antacids. On getting up the next day I still had the indigestion, but started having bowel problems. This went on for two weeks; I felt unwell and couldn't eat. My bowel motions began becoming looser and looser till everything started going right through me. The GP suggested I go on a liquid diet for three or four days, but I lost a stone and felt weaker. I was also suffering from nausea. I had all the tests, and my GP said it was my nervous disposition that was making me ill. I tried everything to get better, but it became worse. I had pain, loss of appetite and eventually depression.'

Some people link their IBS to a period of stress:

'I have always suffered from a "nervous stomach" at times of stress but it went back to normal once the stressful situation had passed. But a little while ago I was off work for four months with various medical problems, and it was all too much for me to cope

2

with. During this time my nervous stomach was completely out of control. The diarrhoea was so bad I couldn't leave the house, I felt very nauseous and had a lot of stomach pain. I also had this most peculiar sensation in my stomach as if there was something alive in there and it was chewing at my insides. I have had all the tests and have been prescribed all sorts of medications, but nothing helps.'

Others are totally puzzled by their IBS, which seems to have come on suddenly, without any warning:

'Mine came on very suddenly. In the night I woke up with severe pains in my stomach and upper abdomen and started being violently sick, with excessive diarrhoea. My GP took me into hospital where they took my gallbladder away, but after the operation I was still suffering very bad pains and still vomiting and having diarrhoea. I lost my job because I was unwell. After eight times in and out of hospital I was told that all I had was IBS. It made me feel that no one believed I was ill because it was made out that it was nothing important.'

'About four years ago when I was 55 diarrhoea started suddenly, and when it didn't clear up I went to the doctor. He gave me tablets but that didn't work. I lost two and a half stone, and was very worried. I pass wind a lot, which is embarrassing and out of control at times.'

'My IBS started just after the war. I tend to have spells of trouble on and off which last from a few days to several months. I never know what really triggers off an attack which comes when I am not stressed or anxious. I do not get bad diarrhoea, mainly looseness or constipation, but I do have a great deal of pain, particularly with the looseness. Also, wind is very troublesome and seems to be the cause of much of the pain. The pain often wakes me at night.'

Some sufferers found that their IBS started after an abdominal operation:

'I have suffered for six years. After a hysterectomy in 1985 I had problems with constipation and severe spasms. It took 12 months of going to the hospital before they told me it was IBS.'

About a quarter of those people suffered with IBS after having gastroenteritis or food poisoning:

'Just over three years ago I suffered food poisoning. This went, but some time after I started to have griping pains and my bowel pattern became irregular – alternate constipation with small pellet motions and then larger motions, sometimes a bit loose, but not really diarrhoea. My stomach rumbled and I started to have bloating and pain, mainly on the left-hand side of the abdomen, with muscle spasm and a feeling of being over-full after a large meal.'

It can be seen that there is no clear pattern in the way IBS starts. In some people the symptoms creep up gradually; in others, they come suddenly after gastroenteritis or a stressful event.

What are the symptoms of IBS?

You can see from the above accounts that IBS is made up of many different symptoms. People classified as having IBS may have some or many of the following problems.

Abdominal pain and spasm
Pain can be experienced throughout the abdomen and in different sites at different times. IBS sufferers usually find the pain is in the lower abdomen, although some also experience it in the upper abdomen. Some people find the pain is worst in the early hours of the morning.

Diarrhoea, constipation, or an alternation of both
In IBS, diarrhoea is caused by food moving too quickly through the system. However, some studies have shown that although transit times tend to be a little faster in those with diarrhoea, the major feature of the diarrhoea is an increased frequency of small amounts of stool. In fact, stool weight per day in IBS patients may be exactly the same as people without IBS – it's just that sufferers with diarrhoea pass motions far more frequently.

'Constipation' means infrequent or difficult bowel movements. Food moves too slowly through the system, so there is too much water absorption and faeces become dry and hard.

People with long-term IBS frequently tell us they no longer know whether their bowel habits are normal or not. Thus, sufferers often worry because they feel they have too many or

4

too few bowel movements. There is in fact a wide variation in the bowel habits of people without IBS – some people go once every three days, some three times a day, and there are many whose bowel habits vary from week to week. It is hard to say what is normal. Bowel habits also depend on the country you are in – by Western criteria all Ugandan villagers have diarrhoea because they produce more than 400 g of unformed stool every day (the Western figure is 300 g per day[1]). Researchers have tried to define constipation and diarrhoea precisely – for instance, some researchers may define constipation as not more than three hard stools per week, with straining, and diarrhoea as more than twenty-one unformed stools per week – but such precise definitions cannot work. Someone who has watery motions and has to get to a toilet urgently may be certain they have diarrhoea, even if their bowel patterns do not strictly conform to the 'over twenty one' criterion.

People who have an alternation of diarrhoea and constipation perhaps find this more difficult to cope with – they never know from one minute to the next how their bowels are going to work, and find it difficult to take medication. Any laxative for constipation may bring on an episode of diarrhoea, and an anti-diarrhoeal drug may cause constipation. This is a difficult problem.

Bloated stomach, rumbling noises and wind

Most sufferers have to put up with the digestive system making loud rumbling noises at random times of the day. Although it is said that other people rarely notice these noises, the people we talked to were very bothered by them. Again, while the average person passes wind 17 times a day without noticing it, IBS sufferers are generally aware that they are passing wind and are worried that other people know too. The embarrassment adds to their other discomforts. Some IBS sufferers also have to wear loose clothes if they suffer from a bloated stomach:

'I cannot fit into any of my clothes, and tend to find that I cannot finish a meal because I feel bloated and full.'

'I am becoming desperate. This condition is so embarrassing. I

5

constantly need to go to the loo and I suffer from terrible bouts of wind, which is so embarrassing. In my job I deal with people all the time so you can imagine how difficult it is. I have to refuse to go out because of it.'

'After having my second child I noticed that I felt bloated and wanted to pass wind, as well as having gurgles and cramps. They came on suddenly after a meal and often I would have to rush to the loo, where I would have very runny motions. As you can appreciate it is very embarrassing, especially if you're in somebody else's house. I would be terrified they would hear me passing wind and I'd be scared to get off the loo in case I had to go back five minutes later.'

'I broke wind one day at work, and someone laughed. I felt so humiliated I felt like walking out.'

Urgency

Once the sufferer has the urge to go to the toilet, he or she has to get there pretty quickly! Sixteen per cent of IBS sufferers have experienced bowel incontinence at some time or another. Most sufferers are very aware of toilets – their life revolves around them, and it is difficult for them to arrange any journey without knowing exactly where the toilets will be situated.

A *feeling of incomplete emptying of the bowels*

Quite often, sufferers will find that they leave the toilet feeling that they have not done all that they could have. Many people find that within a few minutes they have to rush to the toilet again. This may happen three or four times in succession, or even more. Needless to say, this is very disruptive to normal everyday life!

A *sharp pain felt low down inside the rectum*

Attacks can be mild or severe enough to make you almost faint. Luckily, most people find this pain passes off in less than five minutes. This also sometimes happens to people without IBS. The cause of this proctalgia fugax, as it is called, is unknown. Although IBS sufferers are more likely than non-sufferers to get this feeling, it is not one of the more common symptoms.

Nausea, belching and vomiting
Again, these are not common symptoms; although some sufferers experience nausea to a degree which leaves them feeling weak and unable to eat.

How many people have IBS?

Estimates vary as to the number of people who have IBS. Some researchers say it affects 15 per cent of the population in developed countries.[2] Others say that it could be as high as 35 per cent[3]. In any case, IBS accounts for almost half of all consultations to gastroenterologists, making IBS a very expensive complaint – and most gastroenterologists do not feel able to treat patients effectively.

Researchers found symptoms of bowel disorders in over 300 apparently healthy subjects, although few people had bothered to consult a doctor – those seen by physicians are just the tip of the iceberg.[4] People usually go to the GP and receive a diagnosis of IBS when their symptoms become more frequent, or more painful. There are twice as many women as men diagnosed as having IBS in Britain, although this is probably because women in this country tend to go to the doctor more than men anyway. In India the situation is reversed – four times more men than women being diagnosed as having IBS.

In the past it has been difficult to diagnose someone as having IBS; different doctors used different criteria. However, many researchers and doctors now use the Manning Criteria[5]. In 1978 Manning and his team defined IBS as abdominal pain associated with three or more of the following symptoms:

- Pain relieved by defecation.
- More frequent stools with pain onset.
- Looser stools with pain onset.
- Abdominal distension.
- Mucus in the stool.
- Feeling of incomplete evacuation after defecation.

A patient is likely to be diagnosed as having IBS if she or he has pain along with at least three of the above symptoms, and in the absence of any other disease. If you have abdominal pain without any bowel disturbance, and you are told you have IBS, you should question the diagnosis. IBS is a syndrome – that is, a collection of symptoms – and it should not be diagnosed on the basis of only one symptom. In our experience this sometimes happens. If you have constipation only, you are not considered to have IBS.

Symptoms that are not due to IBS

In women
It is sometimes the case that women are diagnosed as having IBS when really their problem is gynaecological. For instance, women have been told they have IBS when they actually have pelvic inflammatory disease (PID) or endometriosis. PID is an inflammation of the pelvic organs which can be due to infection of the fallopian tubes, ovaries, or both. PID can cause a sharp pain throughout the abdomen, although sometimes the pain may be dull. Someone with PID is likely to have other symptoms: pain or bleeding from the vagina during or after intercourse and an abnormal vaginal discharge. Endometriosis is a condition in which parts of the womb lining (endometrial cells) migrate to other organs, for example the bladder or the bowel. These cells act as though they are still in the womb, so they respond every month to the hormones produced during the menstrual cycle – they thicken, enlarge and bleed. This can cause great pain in the abdomen, and sometimes in the back. Intercourse is often extremely painful, periods are heavy as well as painful, and they often become worse towards the end. Because adhesions may have stuck the bowel to the womb, a woman can have bowel symptoms as well. In research carried out by the Endometriosis Society in the USA, nearly three per cent of women subsequently diagnosed as having endometriosis had been previously diagnosed as having IBS.[6] Treating endometriosis frequently brought relief of their gastrointestinal symptoms.

Both PID and endometriosis are treatable. If you have bleeding from the vagina in between periods, if your period pains become worse at the end of the period, if you have an unusual discharge, then insist that you see a gynaecologist. While IBS symptoms are often worse during a menstrual period, IBS does not cause the symptoms mentioned above. Neither should sex be extremely painful! If it is, then do not accept a diagnosis of IBS without seeing a gynaecologist. This is the story of one person wrongly diagnosed as having IBS:

'I had what was called IBS for three years. My main symptom was pain. I did have some bowel problems. I also had bleeding in between periods, and painful sex. My periods were so painful I sometimes fainted. The GP said my symptoms were due to stress. Over the years the pain was sometimes so excruciating I called doctors out or went to casualty. They always told me it was IBS. In the end it was so bad I paid privately for a laparoscopy – they found I had one of the worse cases of endometriosis ever. Once I was cured of the endometriosis, all the "IBS" symptoms disappeared.'

In women and men

Other symptoms which should be checked before IBS is confirmed are rapid loss of weight and rectal bleeding. These are two symptoms which could be due to other more serious diseases. Having said that, however, many people with IBS do lose quite a bit of weight, either because of constant diarrhoea or because of the worry associated with having an illness, especially before it is diagnosed as IBS. Bleeding from the rectum can be due to haemorrhoids or more serious causes, so it is important to go to your GP to have this checked out.

Will IBS lead to cancer?

IBS is not associated with any other disease; it cannot lead to cancer and there are no fatalities. This may be one reason why IBS is not taken seriously. However, IBS is a very common condition which causes misery to hundreds of thousands of people, costs the National Health Service vast sums of money and affects employers whose employees lose time from work. It is therefore important to take IBS as seriously as any other illness.

What sort of people have IBS?

According to research, the average age at which symptoms become apparent is about 29 although the range is about one to 63.[7] However, the people we talked to when we were researching this book ranged from 20 to 78 years. Most were women who had suffered from IBS for anything between 6 months and 50 years! The majority of people, however, had suffered from IBS for less than 10 years. The people we spoke to were of all ages, both sexes, and with all sorts of occupations.

What causes IBS?

IBS can be considered as a disease of function, rather than of structure – in other words, there is nothing physically wrong with any specific part of the digestive system, it is the way the system works that is wrong. IBS has been considered by many practitioners to be a motility disorder (motility meaning movement), that is, the contents of the gut move either too quickly or too slowly through the system. However, the case for IBS being a motility disorder is not really established. Contractile activity in IBS may be quite normal and if it is not, the responses are often exaggerated rather than, strictly speaking, abnormal. IBS is therefore really a disease of exaggerated gut reaction, although this aspect of it may not afflict all patients.

People may be puzzled when they are told they have IBS, as it often comes on suddenly and they can see no good reason for it. The causes of IBS are still largely unknown, and there are no cures which are lastingly effective. While there are various theories as to what causes it, none of them are very satisfactory.

Here we give you a brief outline of the various theories which attempt to explain why people suffer from IBS. These theories are discussed in more detail in the chapters to follow. However, in order to understand the theories fully, it is important to have some knowledge of your digestive system.

Physiology of the gut

The term 'gut' encompasses all of the digestive system, from the mouth to the anus. It thus includes the oesophagus, stomach, small intestine, colon and rectum. The gut has its own nervous system, called the enteric nervous system, the activity of which is modulated by the brain via the autonomic nerves and hormones.

The gut is basically a hollow tube which is made up of smooth muscle tissue that is not under voluntary control. Although some people believe it is only active when you eat, this is not true – the gut is almost always active. It does not, of course, work on its own – it is controlled by the nervous system. This is the system which relays information from the outside and from internal organs to the brain so that it can process this information and act accordingly. The nervous system can be divided into two: the central nervous system (brain and spinal cord) and the peripheral nervous system (which includes the enteric nervous system). Your digestive system is controlled by a complex interaction of these systems, with paths of nerves linking the brain and gut. Your hormonal system also works to keep the gut functioning normally, various circulating hormones exerting powerful effects on the muscle of the gut.

The oesophagus is about 20 cm (8 in) long, and leads from the mouth to the stomach. It secretes mucus and transports food to the stomach. When you eat, food is moved down the oesophagus by an involuntary muscular process called peristalsis in which waves of muscular contractions pass along the length of the ocsophagus. The passage of solid food from the mouth to the stomach takes about six seconds. Once the food is in your stomach it cannot normally pass upwards again; a one-way valve allows food to go downwards only.

The stomach is quite small, but can expand to contain large amounts of food. Food is broken down by various enzymes produced by the stomach, and by mixing and churning movements. This process is controlled by messages conveyed via the nervous system, and by chemical messages (hormones). Peristaltic waves occur in the stomach about three times a minute. Emotions such

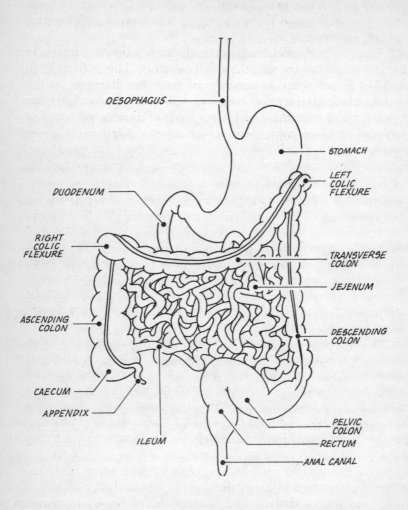

OESOPHAGUS

STOMACH

LEFT
COLIC
FLEXURE

DUODENUM

RIGHT
COLIC
FLEXURE

TRANSVERSE
COLON

JEJENUM

ASCENDING
COLON

DESCENDING
COLON

CAECUM

APPENDIX

PELVIC
COLON

ILEUM

RECTUM

ANAL CANAL

The digestive system, or gut

as anger, fear or anxiety can slow down digestion in the stomach, while excitement speeds up the process. The stomach empties its contents within two to six hours after eating. Carbohydrates pass most quickly through the stomach, proteins are a little slower, and fats are slowest.

When the food has been sufficiently broken down it travels to the next section of the gut, the small intestine. This is 6 m (20 ft) long but is coiled up, as you can see from the diagram. As the food travels down the small intestine, nutrients are absorbed from it through the intestinal walls. Two kinds of movement occur in the small intestine: movements which mix the intestinal contents together, and peristaltic waves which pass the contents along. Intestinal juices secreted for absorption and digestion include pancreatic juices, which contain enzymes that break down proteins, fats and carbohydrates. The material remains in the small intestine for three to five hours, during which time water is reabsorbed from the material into the body. The semi-liquid material is called chyme.

The large intestine, or colon, is about 1.5 m (5 ft) long. Much of the pain associated with IBS is likely to derive from the colon. The nutrients have mostly been absorbed by the time food enters the colon. Waste material is prepared for elimination by the action of bacteria known as the gut flora. These bacteria ferment any remaining carbohydrates and release various gases which contribute to flatulence. The material remains in the large intestine for three to ten hours, and should at this time be solid or semi-solid, as the water from the waste material should have been reabsorbed by this time. Muscular contractions ensure the faeces are pushed along the large bowel to the rectum. Whether they are solid or semi-solid depends on the length of time they are exposed to this process of absorption.

As the rectum (20 cm/8 in long) fills up with waste material, it triggers the urge to expel the faeces. About 100 g (4 oz) of faeces are passed daily, mostly composed of water, inorganic matter, cellulose, fatty substances, mucus and bacteria – the latter comprising 80 per cent of faecal solids. The anal sphincter, which keeps the bowel shut, is under voluntary control and if you relax it the waste material will be allowed out. If the rectum is not emptied it will relax and the desire to defecate will pass.

This is how the normal gut works. It may sound simple, but in fact the process is very complicated. The nervous system of the brain and the gut, and hormones and other chemicals all have to work in harmony if everything is to go according to plan.

Theories of causation

Physiological factors

The brain-gut link The gut has its own nervous system which gastroenterologists sometimes think of as the 'little brain'.[8] This means that is incorrect to think of the gut as being controlled directly by your brain as the gut itself is capable of having some control, although what happens in your gut will be passed through to the 'big brain' in your head and vice versa. Digestive functions are controlled by an interaction between the big brain and the little brain. It could be that IBS is due to a failure in the way the brain-gut relationship functions.

Disorder of the smooth muscle tissue It has been suggested that some IBS patients may have hyper-reactive, or oversensitive, bowel muscle. This could be genetically determined (inherited), or it could be acquired (for instance from an attack of gastro-enteritis[9]). According to this theory, IBS could be a disorder of the smooth muscle tissue. Being born with such a disorder, or acquiring it later in life, would mean that you are likely to get IBS, which could be triggered by factors such as some types of food, stress, or hormone abnormalities. People without the underlying abnormality of the smooth muscle tissue would not get IBS even when the same triggers were present. People with IBS often have bladder problems such as the need to pass water very frequently. This would tie in with the above theory, as the bladder is also made up of smooth muscle tissue.

New techniques of measuring motility in the gut (the speed at which digested food is moved along) have shown that there are abnormalities in the electrical pattern in the gut in some people with IBS; these abnormalities can be triggered by stress or certain drugs, but they are also present without triggering factors. For instance, researchers recorded gut movements while people played computer games, drove in London traffic, and heard their own voices through headphones.[10] These activities are acknowledged as being stressful. One or more abnormalities was seen in 19 out of 22 IBS patients, but only one in ten non-IBS people. This leads to the conclusion that IBS sufferers have hyper-reactive bowels which react more to any sort of stress than those of normal people.

Fatty meals have also been shown to provoke a different pattern of motor activity (movements) in the small intestines of IBS patients.

Other researchers measured motor activity in the small intestines of people going about their own business (i.e. not doing specific tasks set by the researchers).[11] These studies found that there were differences in the motor activity in the gut between IBS sufferers and healthy people. It is possible that the disturbed motility produces the symptoms of distension, discomfort, and an inappropriate urge to go to the toilet.

Professor Read, Professor of Gastrointestinal Physiology and Nutrition at The University of Sheffield Northern General Hospital, explains that some people have an oversensitive rectum, which makes them feel as if they need to go to the toilet when physically there really is no need.[12] Some people may have the opposite problem; they may have an undersensitive rectum so that they do not realize when they need to go, leading to constipation. Professor Read also states that some people suffer from an oversensitive or undersensitive bowel, not just the rectum, and believes that most people with IBS can be placed in one of these categories.

Sometimes people blame themselves for having IBS – 'If only I could cope better with stress,' they say, or 'I realize I have to control it with my mind'. Often they feel guilty because they still have the symptoms even when they are leading a relatively stress-free life. They may feel that there is something wrong with them if they cannot control their symptoms. This is why it is important for you to know that there is evidence that the tendency to have IBS is biological. That is to say, you have a predisposition to IBS, and there is nothing you can do about that!

Genetic predisposition There is some debate about whether the predisposition to IBS is inherited. One study has shown that symptoms are more likely to develop when there is an abnormality in the automatic nervous system, which makes the gut more susceptible to sudden changes in blood flow.[13] Such increases in blood flow are associated with attacks of pain. A disorder of the autonomic nervous system also gives rise to migraines, and it has been found that families of IBS patients have a higher rate of migraine headaches. This gives support to the view that IBS might be due to a dysfunction of the autonomic nervous system, and that such dysfunction might be inherited. However, the study was conducted on people with recurrent abdominal pain, which may or may not have been IBS.

Trigger factors

A response to stress The colon normally moves food by moderate contractions or spasms. If a person with IBS becomes excited or anxious the colon reacts with either too few or too many contractions, leading to either constipation or diarrhoea. The trigger factor theory accepts that there could be a predisposition to IBS, either hereditary or acquired, and that stress of any kind acts as a trigger. Consequently counselling or stress control could be of benefit. Stress is covered in more detail in Chapter 6.

Dietary factors It used to be thought that IBS was due to too little fibre in the diet. Fibre decreases the transit time and also the reabsorption of water from the faeces in the colon. This increases the volume of the faeces, makes them pass more easily through the colon, and also results in increased frequency of defecation. However, since IBS people do not differ from non-IBS people in their intake of fibre, this is not now thought to be the cause of IBS. See Chapter 6 for more information on diet.

Many people feel that certain foods make their IBS worse. This is not the same as saying that these foods cause IBS. Although some researchers feel that food intolerance can cause IBS, this is not the consensus of medical opinion. However, certain foods could act as a trigger, setting off an attack of IBS in people already predisposed to it.

Hysterectomy A recent study attempted to find out whether hysterectomy patients have an increased risk of IBS. [14] Symptoms were measured in over 200 women six weeks before, and then again six months after, their operation. One in five women had symptoms of IBS (mostly the constipation type) before their operation, and over half these women actually improved after their hysterectomy. However, one in five women had increased symptoms. One in ten women who had been symptom-free before their operation showed signs of IBS afterwards, most of these cases being constipation-predominant IBS.

The researchers concluded that many women who already have symptoms when they go for hysterectomy improve afterwards, but some women who have no IBS symptoms beforehand can be expected to have IBS problems later. It seems that hysterectomy can act as a trigger for IBS in some women, but it is not known why this is.

Another study found that women who had had a hysterectomy were more likely to have constipation than other women. [15] This is thought to be because altered hormone concentration may affect bowel habit after hysterectomy, especially in women who have also had their ovaries removed. It is also possible that the operation on the pelvic area may have caused damage to the nerves in that region.

Gall bladder trouble Some of the people we spoke to said their IBS began after their gall bladders were removed. According to Professor Read, this can give rise to IBS because the bile acid can leak into the duodenum, and if it is not absorbed it can have a laxative effect. A 'faulty' gall bladder can provoke the same response. [16]

Mercury poisoning Some people believe that IBS can be triggered by mercury poisoning. Roger Dyson, a homeopath, has studied the work of homeopath Pritam Singh and some of the writings of J. G. Levenson, President of the British Dental Society for Clinical Nutrition. Roger Dyson now believes that mercury (used for filling teeth) gives off a vapour which, when swallowed, combines with hydrochloric acid to form mercuric chloride; this destroys gut bacteria and allows an overgrowth of candida. The formation of this compound may leave the body deficient in hydrochloric acid so that digestion cannot proceed efficiently. Roger Dyson says that the effects of mercury poisoning can be slow, taking maybe five years or more to show. Why doesn't everyone with mercury fillings, then, have the symptoms of IBS? Dyson says that some people are more resilient than others, and not everyone is sensitive to the effects of mercury. According to Dyson, you do not need to rush to the dentist to have your fillings out – homeopathic remedies may, he says, help this condition. [17]

Hormones Oestrogen and progesterone affect the function of the colon and the movement of food through it. There are some women whose symptoms fluctuate with the menstrual cycle, which is governed by these hormone. However, this is not likely to be a major contributory factor in IBS – although twice as many women as men are diagnosed as having IBS in Britain, this is not the case in other countries. It is possible, though, that these hormones can worsen IBS at certain times of the month for some women.

Disturbance of gut flora The balance of different bacteria in the gut can be altered by taking antibiotics, or by a bout of gastroenteritis. Some researchers believe that IBS may be a result of the gut flora becoming disturbed – the 'good' bacteria get pushed out, allowing the 'bad' bacteria or yeasts (such as candida) to take over. You will find more about this in Chapter 6.

Psychological factors
Many studies find IBS patients to be more anxious and depressed than non-IBS patients. Some researchers have concluded that their IBS is thus due to anxiety and depression. (See Chapter 6 for more on this.) In other words, IBS occurs as a result of the psychological disorder. At the moment there is no way of knowing whether this is the case, or whether having a disorder like IBS causes the anxiety and depression.

A particular type of personality? To find out whether IBS sufferers have a distinct personality, scientific studies have concentrated on comparing them with other groups of patients such as sufferers of Crohn's disease. Both groups are tested on psychological measures such as neuroticism, extroversion, hostility, fatigue, depression, anxiety and so on, and differences between the groups are compared. Studies sometimes contradict each other, but IBS patients do tend to be more anxious than other people. However, no distinctive personality type has yet been pinpointed. Dr Paul Latimer, a professor of psychiatry in the USA, says: 'Psychological studies have found patients to be compulsive, over-conscientious, dependent, sensitive, guilty and unassertive.' 'Little evidence exists that IBS patients have a distinctive personality profile.'[18] Other studies have come to the same conclusion.[19]

Can IBS be cured?

There is nothing that cures all the symptoms of IBS, but there are various treatments which can ease some of them. People do recover from IBS. You can help yourself by finding out as much as possible about IBS, including the theories of how IBS starts, and what treatments are available. Self-help groups are very useful because sufferers feel less alone and more in control of themselves and their symptoms, and they often pick up tips on useful treatments. In the following chapters we will describe the medical investigations IBS sufferers undergo, the various treatments, and the physical and psychological consequences of having IBS. We will also look at how IBS sufferers cope with the condition, and the roles played by stress and lifestyle. The people quoted in this book all suffer, or have suffered, from IBS. It is to be hoped that their stories of how they coped will help you understand IBS and be able to deal with the disorder more effectively.

Chapter 2

Testing Time: Medical Investigations

'Doctors are not used to helping, just diagnosing.'

This chapter will discuss what to expect when you decide that you need help for your IBS symptoms and the tests you may have to undergo, although not exactly pleasant, are not as bad as you may imagine. Our studies show that people who have information on medical investigations find them less stressful than do those who do not know what is going to happen; they are less anxious and therefore cope better.

Most people with symptoms of IBS go to their GP, although they may of course have tried to treat themselves with laxatives, anti-diarrhoeal mixtures or indigestion remedies. As we have seen, the symptoms of IBS are common in the general population, almost a third of whom have experienced such symptoms at some time in their lives. In fact, one study found that one or more symptoms occurred frequently in nearly fifty per cent of women and twenty-five per cent of men![1] However, IBS as diagnosed by doctors is present in one in ten women and one in twenty men. People put up with these symptoms for four to five years before going to their doctor. Why do people wait so long? And why do some people seek help from the medical profession while others do not? Some researchers have suggested that the sufferers who go to the doctors with their symptoms are more psychologically disturbed than those who do not, although their symptoms may be the same as those who do not seek help.[2] However, the researchers found that the more symptoms people had, the more likely they were to consult their doctor (not surprisingly!). They were more likely to seek help for their abdominal pain rather than the other symptoms of IBS. The researchers concluded that IBS is very prevalent in the general population, especially in women, and that the factors that made some people consult their doctors, joining the ranks of the 'IBS patients', were the number and intensity of their symptoms.

We all know that there are wide-ranging symptoms involved in IBS. Some of us have many symptoms, others have fewer. All of the symptoms of IBS are hard to deal with, but, as in the study above, the people we talked to also stated that abdominal pain was the problem that made them seek help. People also mentioned that as a consequence of IBS they slept less, and were therefore more tired.

What happens when you go to the doctor?

Some GPs diagnose IBS without any tests at all; this is more likely to happen if the sufferer is young, and fit apart from the symptoms of IBS.

The GP is likely to feel your abdomen, and, if you are a woman, give you a gynaecological examination to make sure the problem really is to do with the gut. You will be asked to undress from the waist down and lie on the couch with your knees raised. A blanket will probably be put over you, for the sake of modesty. The doctor will put on a pair of gloves and insert his or her fingers into the vagina in order to feel for abnormalities. A swab may be taken. This will be cultured in a laboratory to test for certain bacteria. The results are likely to show there is nothing abnormal.

The next test may be a rectal examination. This time you will lie on your left-hand side and bend your knees (the left-hand side is always used simply to ensure consistency in doctor's findings). The doctor will put on some gloves and, using a lubricant, insert his or her fingers into the anus, feeling the rectum. You may find this unpleasant, but it is not actually painful.

The doctor may take some blood or send you to hospital for a blood test and ask you for a urine sample and for a stool sample to send off for analysis. The blood tests will show whether you are anaemic or not, and whether inflammation is present. These results will be normal for most IBS patients. The stool sample will show whether you are bleeding, or whether there are parasites in the stools. Again, for most people these results will be normal. The doctor will then either send you for hospital tests, or make a diagnosis of IBS on the spot.

From our experience we can say that most of you will find your GP treats you fairly well, and with sympathy:

'My own GP was very sympathetic and he is pleased to discuss my problems with me anytime.'

He recommended a high-fibre diet, and experimenting with bran and medication, and added that it was very difficult to treat.'

'My doctor is always sympathetic and listens to me. She's very nice, although there's nothing she can do for the pain or the other symptoms. I've been going to her every few months for three years now. She may think I'm neurotic but she never shows it anyway!'

However, about a quarter of the people who spoke to us felt that their GP did not understand their problems, and was not sympathetic.

'As if he thought I was making it all up to get out of going to school and didn't believe me.' (*Pauline, a schoolgirl at the time of diagnosis, has had IBS for 27 years*).

'As if I were neurotic and needed a tranquillizer.' (*A 58-year-old woman, 38 at time of diagnosis.*)

'He did his best, but he didn't really understand how devastatingly embarrassing it was for a girl just growing up. I felt unattractive because of it.' (*Andrea, 14 years old at the time*).

'In 1966 GPs did not do so many tests. He said, "Go home and have a cup of coffee, it will calm you down."'

'The first doctor laughed – then advised bran.'

'I lost two stone in three weeks (reaching six stone) and he just gave me an anti-diarrhoeal drug and said he'd see me in another week.'

'I was given anti-depression tablets and told it was all in my mind and to go away and sort myself out.'

23

'They were patronizing – why don't you go and have a holiday? Didn't treat me with any urgency as though just because I didn't have a recognized or terminal illness I couldn't be in much pain.'

'I was frightened to go back because he just dismisses me as neurotic, but recently I've had to go back because it's become so chronic. I'm signed off work for two months now.'

'I do find the doctors are not very sympathetic about this complaint and never seem to talk about it as an illness. They regard it as something we have to live with. I think if a few of them had it badly, they might go out of their way to find a cure.'

Indeed, some people may consider changing their GP because they do not feel they have been taken seriously. If you are one of these people, and you find your GP is not treating you as you would wish, then do not suffer in silence. Explain to your GP just how your symptoms are affecting you. Ask to be taken seriously and perhaps show your doctor some literature on IBS – many doctors do not keep up with the latest research and still believe IBS reflects a neurotic personality. Even if this were the case, you still deserve to be treated properly! If your doctor is really unhelpful, though, consider changing to another practice. Although this will be a bother for you, IBS can affect you over a fairly long period and having a sympathetic doctor whom you can trust and talk to with confidence can really help you through this time. Although you cannot expect to be cured, you have a right to be treated with respect and sympathy. If you need to change your doctor, do so, but you must choose carefully – you do not want to change your doctor to one who is no more helpful.

Hospital tests

As there are no positive tests for IBS, investigations are done to reassure the patient and physician that the patient has no serious disease. Thompson says that tests should not be conducted without serious thought, because they quite often produce results which are contradictory and, if repeatedly done, may undermine the patient's confidence in the diagnosis of IBS.[3]

McCloy and McCloy also feel that hospital investigations are not necessary to make the diagnosis of IBS.[4] However, they say that IBS is rare after 60 years of age, and that any elderly patient who goes to their GP with IBS-like symptoms and weight loss should be investigated by hospital tests. They feel that hospital investigations are distressing to the patient, who undergoes one negative test after another and feels more and more as if they are regarded as a fraud. They say that the approach of excluding all serious diseases leads to hospital doctors dismissing the patients as neurotic once all the tests have been found negative. Carol says:

'I have suffered considerable discomfort and pain for almost 10 years now. I have had all manner of tests and X-rays, all with a negative result. This year I had a test under general anaesthetic to see if I have coeliac disease. However, again this proved negative and the consultant I had been visiting discharged me, saying he could only put the problem down to IBS. I find all this really stressful.'

According to Deidre:

'When the results of barium X-rays indicate to the gastroenter-ologist that there is an abnormality of the bowels, then he or she should be in a position to do something for you rather than saying that you have IBS and to go back and see your GP to prescribe you medicine. I had a barium meal and enema in 1989 followed by a further one recently as my pain had considerably worsened and my GP felt that a further test was well overdue. After my last visit to the gastroenterologist I was no wiser, and actually felt it all to have been a waste of time. I feel, however, that the attitude of my GP is one of sympathy with this condition and I have never been given the cold shoulder but have been prescribed with a variety of medicines. There is little else to suggest as the barium X-rays indicate IBS and at least a clean bill of health – there's no cancer or anything.'

McCloy and McCloy say that there are far too many tests, they cost the NHS vast amounts of money, and they mean both distress and risks to the patient. They want there to be positive criteria for diagnosing IBS, rather than diagnosis by exclusion. However, many doctors are cautious, knowing that if they do not send patients to hospital to exclude more serious diseases, IBS, may be a misdiagnosis. McCloy and McCloy show that this is unlikely to happen, but it is a possibility. Some people who are told they probably have IBS no doubt want the tests, for they are themselves worried that they may have a more serious disease:

'I had a range of tests performed – these included a barium enema, a lactose tolerance test and a sigmoidoscopy. The tests were negative, but what really concerned me is that my father contracted rectal cancer when he was in his fifties and had to have a colostomy. Then the cancer spread to his liver and he died. My father's early symptoms were very similar to my own.'

'I have recently been diagnosed as having IBS, after lots of different tests, e.g. endoscopy, gall bladder tests, X-rays, dilation and curettage (a gynaecological procedure), laparoscopy etc; these all proved negative. My GP told me it was all in the mind, but the hospital doctor said IBS is now being recognized as an illness. At times I thought there must be something seriously wrong with me, because my mother died of cancer; this was the first thing I thought of.'

The following is one woman's medical history since contracting IBS consisting of many tests, all showing nothing seriously wrong. As you read it, you may feel that it is not worth going through all these tests, if you are young and, apart from IBS, healthy:

8.8.85 Codeine phosphate prescribed.
13.9.85 Consultant prescribes eight-day course of flagyl for suspected giardiasis (antibiotic for parasites thought to be in gut).
25.9.85 Radiodiagnosis washout and barium enema (no abnormalities).
4.11.85 Samples of stools over three days (for parasites).
18.11.85 Blood test and three more days of stool samples.
9.12.85 Blood test.
16.12.85 Gall bladder X-ray
18.12.85 Blood test for thyroid deficiency.
19.12.85 Further ultrasound (nothing shows up).
13.1.86 Barium meal X-ray (all clear).
11.2.86 Smear test (all clear).
16.4.86 More blood tests.
7.5.86 Thyroid uptake scan for thyrotoxicosis (all OK).
15.5.86 Stool samples over three days.
16.5.86 Barium enema.
21.5.86 Results of tests and scan all OK; no blood in stools. Diagnosis is giardiasis.

23.6.86 Still thinks it's giardiasis. Blood test and three more stool tests.

30.6.86 No sign of giardiasis in stools, but given eight more days of flagyl.

25.7.86 Gastroenterologist suggests it could be pancreas inefficiency: I have now lost two stone in weight, blood test for red cell folate.

31.7.86 X-ray – small bowel enema.

19.8.86 One swallow test. Tube and crosby capsule X-rays and gastric juices test.

1.9.86 Endoscopy: all OK.

10.9.86 Not coeliac disease or giardiasis.

1.10.8 Diagnosis: body making too much bacteria. Four weeks antibiotics.

4.9.90 Overall blood test (result normal).

'Result: IBS.

This is another woman's experience of her symptoms and the tests that were conducted:

'I consulted my GP in February 1991 for lower abdominal pain, and pain on passing urine. The doctor said it could be appendicitis or a urine infection, and to send in a urine specimen, but to call her if the pain became worse. It did become worse; I couldn't walk; she did a home visit and I was referred to the hospital. I was sent up to a ward where the doctor examined my abdomen, took some blood and said there was nothing wrong and sent me straight home. Over the weeks the pain got worse – it felt as though something was going to burst inside me. When I had my period the pain worsened. My husband had to call the GP who saw me and referred me to the hospital, where I was admitted. I was told that I probably had a urine infection, a specimen was sent and came back negative; they said that although it was negative it was still probably a urine infection. I had blood taken and a scan was ordered, but this was clear. The pain was getting easier. Then one morning it was extremely severe, and the doctor who saw me ordered an injection of pethidine. Another doctor saw me and said they were referring me to a gynaecologist; I was discharged and told I would receive the appointment in the post.

'I was at home for a while, in pain but trying to tell myself there was nothing wrong. I then had to call the GP out again as the pain was unbearable. I was referred to a gynaecologist and admitted to the hospital, where I was told I probably had a pelvic infection. They took swabs. After this I was put on two courses of antibiotics and discharged. Then I experienced unbearable pain. I was very frightened so went back to the ward I had been in. I was told it was appendicitis or an ectopic pregnancy. A specimen of urine was taken and I was given an injection for the pain. I was told that I would be going to theatre, then I was told it would be the following day. All I wanted was for somebody to find out what the pain was and to stop it. The next day came and I was prepared for theatre, but the morning went and the afternoon came and I still hadn't gone to theatre. The doctor eventually came to tell me that I would be going to theatre that evening for a laparoscopy. When I came out of the anaesthetic I asked the nurse what was wrong. She said everything was clear. That was a relief, but what was causing my pain? The next day I was discharged.

'Days later the pain was still there, and my husband called the GP out. This GP said he thought it could be something to do with my bowel and referred me for an urgent appointment to a gastroenterologist. I saw this doctor within a week. He ordered a barium meal and told me to take Colofac. I had the barium meal, which was negative. I went to my GP for the results, he said everything was fine and that it was IBS. I asked what could be done; he said "Nothing, it's due to stress," and that was that. I felt then that I had wasted everybody's time and that some GPs' attitude is that it is stress and so you as the individual can control it. I don't think that people who have never suffered from this realize how it can affect your life. I know it's not a disease and is only a condition, but I think that GPs should start to recognize it and not just dismiss it or the individual. I have never been back to my doctor about my IBS, I just keep getting repeat prescriptions of Colofac. I want to be able to relax and to control my condition, but on occasions the pain is unbearable still.'

Should you take the tests?

Whether you undergo tests or not depends on the circumstances. If you are at all worried that you might have cancer or some other serious disorder, the tests will put your mind at rest. Dr Chris Mallinson, consultant at Lewisham Hospital, says: 'If you have a patient whose symptoms have lasted a long time and who is still in the early twenties, who has the typical IBS picture and who obeys the doctors' ideas of the Manning criteria, it's perfectly reasonable not to do the tests. However, if you've got someone who is over 40, and whose symptoms are new and rather well localized, then there's no getting away from the tests, however convinced you may be [that it's IBS].'6

Dr Mallinson says that if people start having IBS when they are, say, 50, then a doctor would be taking substantial risks not to recommend taking some tests. Although it is possible for IBS to start at this age it is unusual, and it is at this age that the risk of other diseases increases. Cancer is the big worry, of course, although it is much more likely the person has diverticulosis. (This is when the muscles of the colon wall have become weakened, and have lost their elasticity. Pouches called diverticula are then formed, which may become infected.) Tests would normally eliminate these possibilities. Despite the advice from experts, some of our older members who were in their sixties and seventies at the time of diagnosis were told they had IBS without any tests at all. We suggest that if you are over 50 and your doctor does not refer you for tests, you should ask for them just for safety's sake.

What the tests look for

Tests can detect ulcers (persistent breaches in the skin that will not heal), and patches of inflammation as in Crohn's disease. The latter causes inflammation of the intestines which gives rise to symptoms similar to those of IBS; sometimes the affected part of the intestine has to be removed surgically. Polyps (benign tumours which can lead to cancer), malignant tumours and diverticula can also be detected.

Which tests are conducted depends on the symptoms. If the patient has lower abdominal pains, erratic bowels and tenderness of the left side the first test indicated is a barium enema because this investigation examines the lower part of the guts. If the pain is higher up and there is not much bowel upset the doctor may suspect something is wrong with the small intestine, in which case a barium meal and follow through (see p. 31) may be indicated first as this shows the upper part of the gut. If the patient has symptoms very high up in the gut an endoscopy may be performed, which shows the doctor if there is any abnormality from the throat to the stomach. If there are many different symptoms, as in IBS, the doctor may recommend several checks for certain patients to be on the safe side, for example a barium enema, a barium meal and a scan. If a patient has sharp pains in the chest area which get worse with exercise, the doctor may even want to check the heart with a cardiograph. If the patient complaints of pains in the back, sides and abdomen, a kidney X-ray may be recommended.

Why do people worry about tests?

Quite often IBS sufferers feel that there must be something seriously wrong. This is a natural fear when you are in a lot of pain, have disturbed bowel habits and may have lost weight. Doctors, of course, find that most people who have tests have nothing seriously wrong with them, so they are sometimes indifferent to your fears. However, some IBS patients may have had relatives with bowel cancer, or have had serious medical problems before IBS symptoms began, so it is understandable that they worry. It is important to remember that for the vast majority of people with IBS symptoms the tests will be straightforward and there will be nothing seriously wrong.

Some people may be worried because they fear pain or embarrassment, or think they will feel undignified. However, if you are well informed about the tests, you will be prepared for them; your anxiety level will be lessened, and the tests should not then cause much discomfort. Most tests do not hurt, but anxiety can cause you to tense all your muscles, which makes investigations like barium enemas painful. If you can relax, you will be all right.

Routine tests

The first thing the doctor is likely to do is to feel the abdominal area, and then carry out a sigmoidoscopy. A very straight, narrow tube is inserted into the rectum and pushed as far as possible (different people can tolerate different lengths). The doctor looks through the instrument to detect cancer of the rectum, piles, fissures and cracks in the rectal wall. With the sigmoidoscope, the doctor can examine the lowest part of the bowel; it reaches the parts that the barium enema cannot reach. The patient lies on the left side, with the knees up. Although it can be painful, the pain passes as soon as the instrument is withdrawn.

'It was like having your ears pierced – by the time you realized it was painful, the pain was gone.'

'It was a bit unnerving to have to lie there with doctors looking at my backside, but I was pleased to have the test because I wanted to make sure nothing serious was wrong.'

You can be told the results of this test immediately. The usual result is that nothing abnormal was found.

Barium meal and follow through

Barium is a thick liquid consisting of barium sulphate. The liquid is either swallowed or injected into the rectum. The liquid is radiopaque (opaque to X-rays) and casts shadows on a film. X-ray pictures can show any abnormalities. The meal is insoluble, which means that none of the substance will be absorbed from the intestine.

You will have to do without food for some hours before the barium meal. Swallowing barium (a thick white drink which doctors jocularly refer to as a 'milk shake') makes the digestive tract become opaque. The barium (which has not got an unpleasant taste) moves down the digestive system and is recorded. The X-ray pictures detect ulcers and tumours in the upper part of the digestive tract.

'The doctors and nurses were very nice – joking and laughing with me. They asked me to drink a white milkshake, quite a lot of it. It didn't really taste of anything, but the texture was sort of gooey and chalky. Then I had to lie down on a stretcher for a while. They fetched me into the X-ray room and took a few pictures. Then I had to drink another pint or so of the liquid, wait a while, and then have more pictures taken. It went on for ages. There was nothing painful or embarrassing about this test – it was all quite boring. It took about an hour and a half, and they told me there and then there was nothing wrong.'

Barium enema

The colon must be empty before the barium enema is carried out. This usually means drinking only fluids for a set time before the enema, and taking laxatives the day before. A tube-like instrument is inserted into the rectum (this should not hurt if you relax), and barium flows into the large bowel; air is also pumped into the bowel, which you may find uncomfortable. The pictures of the bowel are transferred on to a monitor – often you can watch what is happening on the screen. The barium enema can detect tumours or inflammation. Most people find the test unpleasant but not particularly painful. Shirley, aged 37:

'I was given a sheet telling me what to do before the test. About two days before I could only eat a low residue diet – fish, eggs, I can't remember what else. Then the day before, just fluids or clear soup. Also the night before I had to take some sort of laxative to clear out the bowel. I was having so much diarrhoea at the time, going to the toilet up to 15 times a day, that the laxatives didn't make any difference anyway. When I went to the hospital the doctor asked me if the laxatives had given me diarrhoea. He didn't look as if he believed me when I said they had made no difference. Then I had to lie on the bed while an instrument was inserted into the rectum. This didn't hurt at all, but when they started pumping air into me I found it quite painful, rather like having bad wind. The white fluid was also pumped up inside, and I could see the fluid flowing through the bowel on the screen. It was quite interesting. Pictures were taken while I was lying down and standing up. The tests were negative. The whole procedure was quite quick. Afterwards, the doctor said to drink plenty of water because the barium would make me constipated. After six months of diarrhoea, I was looking forward to a change!'

Afterwards, you can expect to have flatulence and to keep feeling as if you need to go to the toilet – but it's only air and barium. It can take up to three days to get rid of the barium, during which time your stools are white and don't flush away very easily.

Colonoscopy

This is a more comprehensive test and is conducted in hospital under general anaesthetic. The colonoscope (again, a tube-like instrument) is inserted into the back passage. The doctor looks through a viewer attached to the colonoscope. This test will show up patches of inflammation, as in Crohn's disease, and is the most sensitive way of finding polyps. It also discovers tumours and diverticula. The colonoscope does everything a barium enema can do, and can discover certain things an enema can miss such as small polyps. If polyps are found they can be removed at the time.

For this test the bowel must be empty. It is not the test of first choice, as it takes longer and is more expensive than a barium meal and enema. As this test is usually done under general anaesthetic, no-one wrote to us with an account of their colonoscopy!

Endoscopy

An endoscope is used to relay pictures from the upper part of the digestive tract. An instrument is placed in the throat and the patient swallows it, along with the attached cables. (The throat is first numbed by the use of an anaesthetic spray or, alternatively the patient may be given a general anaesthetic; in either case it is necessary to go without food and drink for some hours beforehand.) The doctor then injects air into the stomach, which inflates it, thus allowing the doctor to see more easily. A biopsy can be performed if necessary.

A 62-year-old woman wrote:

'The specialist came and told us that six of us were due to have the same test. He told us he would be inserting a tube about the size of a fountain pen down our throats and would then take it down into our stomachs and have a look around. He said not to worry that we would not be able to breathe – we would still breathe normally. We had two choices: we could have an anaesthetic or we could opt to have it done without, in which case we would have our throats sprayed to make them numb and then swallow the tube. I asked how many people opted for it this way, and he said just over fifty per cent. It was explained to us that if we had the general anaesthetic we wouldn't know anything that was happening, but of course we would feel tired afterwards. Without the anaesthetic there would be no after-effects, and if we found difficulty in swallowing the tube we could then still have the anaesthetic. It sounded a bit gruesome, but we did not have to decide until the last minute.

'The first lady went in and came back about ten minutes later saying, "Look at me, I'm still alive! It wasn't so bad and I didn't have the anaesthetic." The second lady was away much longer as she had the anaesthetic, and when she came back, was still half- asleep in the chair. Then came my turn. I said I'd be brave and not have a general anaesthetic. I was given a throat spray which tasted a little bitter and then a plastic gadget to keep my teeth apart. I was at this stage lying on my side – I did not have to undress. The doctor came in and gave my throat another spray, and took the tube and told me to feel it with my tongue. The next thing I was being asked to swallow, which I did and was given every encouragement. Then again I was asked to swallow, which made me retch a bit, and again a third time. I was then told the tube was in my stomach and they would now have a look around. The doctor said I could have a look on the video screen and see what was happening. I declined, but have been sorry ever since, as I am sure I would have been very interested. In no time at all it was over, and apart from a slight numbness in the throat it was no trouble at all. The numbness wore off after 20 minutes. We weren't pressurized at all in our choice. I think the doctor's chat to us together at the start was very helpful, as we all were able to talk to each other and give each other encouragement.'

Ultrasound scan

This is the technique used on women who are pregnant. There are said to be no risks attached to it. Sound waves penetrate the body, casting shadows on the video screen. The scan will show up gallstones, fibroids, or any other abnormalities in the abdominal region. You must have a full bladder for this test. It is quite painless, as our respondents describe:

'It was interesting. I had to drink two pints of water before I went and nothing to eat after nine o'clock the previous evening. I was dying to go to the loo, but you have to have a full bladder, or the picture doesn't show up. Luckily they took me straight in! They rubbed a small box over me [a probe] which showed up pictures on the screen. I couldn't make sense of the pictures, but obviously they could. It didn't hurt a bit.'

'No, it didn't hurt, but it was a pain! I got there, full of fluids and feeling uncomfortable, and they were running about an hour late. I couldn't wait – rushed to the loo. What a relief. Then of course when I went in they sent me out again, because the picture wasn't clear as I didn't have any water in my bladder. So I had to sit there for over an hour and a half drinking constantly. I had visions of them being late again, and having to go to the loo again, but it was OK. They didn't find anything abnormal.'

Intravenous urogram

One female respondent had a kidney X-ray called an intravenous urogram. This is not a routine test for patients with IBS symptoms but it is carried out on some. Compounds of iodine are injected into the arm. These are also radiopaque, and cast shadows of the kidneys on to film. We give this account here just in case some of you are sent for it:

'The worse bit was all this purging of the bowel before the X-ray. I'd already done it for the barium enema, so I wasn't looking forward to it again. Two days before the X-ray, I had to take a bottle of laxative – it acted very quickly and very violently. I was on the loo most of the evening, and it was very painful. The strange thing is that the next day I was allowed to eat! I would rather have gone two days without eating than having to have this violent laxative. Anyway, the next day I had to take two Sennacot which didn't appear to do anything. On the day of the X-ray I went in straight away, and the doctor introduced himself and his nurse. They were very pleasant. They explained what was going to happen in detail, in a reassuring manner. They injected a substance, which was a dye, into my arm, and about a minute after it was injected I came over all hot as if I were going to faint, but luckily they had told me to expect this reaction, so I didn't mind. The feeling passed really quickly, then I just lay on the bed while they took the pictures. I had to get up and go to the loo, and then come back for more pictures. They had told me to expect to be there over an hour, but because everything was normal, it only took half an hour. So I went to all that trouble of taking laxatives for nothing. Still, at least I knew I was OK.'

Test results

The staff at the hospital will normally tell you that they have found nothing seriously wrong. It is usually up to your GP to tell you what this means – that is, that you have irritable bowel syndrome. You are probably going to have mixed feelings about the results of the tests. If they are negative (and for a diagnosis of IBS they will be), you will feel relieved on the one hand (thank goodness it's not cancer!) and annoyed on the other, because there is nothing to treat. You may find you feel guilty, as though you are a fraud and have wasted the doctors' time, because there was nothing wrong with you. However, you have *not* wasted anyone's time.

Most hospital tests performed are 'negative', and a good thing too. If your doctor suspected IBS he or she will be expecting the results to be negative, and both of you will feel relieved that they are so. After all, although IBS is very unpleasant it will probably improve, unlike more serious diseases. Also, in having excluded things like cancer and Crohn's disease you now have a diagnosis of IBS, which is better than living with the uncertainty of not knowing what is the matter with you. These are some of the responses you may have when you are told about the results:

'I suppose relieved but at the same time I would like to have been given some hope of anything to take away this pain and improve my way of life . . . I could not believe after six months of waiting the best they could suggest was to take laxatives.'

'Initially relieved, but fed up as it got no better.'

'I expected it but I felt a sense of hopelessness at first, followed quite soon by a determination that it wouldn't defeat me.'

'Pleased, although I felt that was the end of the line and now there was no more treatment available that was likely to be effective.'

As you are reading this book, at least you know about IBS. Some people were totally perplexed when they were told they had IBS as they had never heard of it. It is to be hoped that you will have more help than the following sufferer:

'I wanted to know more but could find no information anywhere. I sought help from a trained nurse, who hadn't heard of it either.'

If your GP is sympathetic you should not have the problems of some sufferers who were informed that they should be able to cure themselves. Some people were told directly that IBS was self-induced, and that if only they could learn to deal with stress or food habits their IBS would improve:

'In 1976 it was called spastic colon. I thought that if I gave up work I would be free of stress, so I retired. The IBS has not improved.'

'The doctor said it was "due to years of bad eating", which I consider impertinent and probably not true.'

'It was put down to exam nerves, then premarital nerves, then postmarital nerves . . . then change of water etc . . .'

'It wasn't explained to me . . . the doctor dismissed it and didn't recognize the problems it was causing me.'

'The tests were very worrying as I feared cancer – I was very relieved when told it was diverticulosis [later IBS was diagnosed] of which I'd never heard. The doctor said it was due to too much Devon cream, which I don't eat.' (*IBS sufferer living in Devon*).

'I was disappointed because I was told it was just my nerves and to go away and eat lots of fibre (with dire results).'

A couple of people suspected their symptoms were IBS:

'I had to tell him [the GP] I had IBS . . . my GP looked doubtful and the specialist said there was no such condition.'

Keeping yourself – and your doctor – informed

If you go for any of these tests, make sure you are kept informed about what is going on at every stage. You should know what the test is for, how long it is going to last, whether it will be painful or uncomfortable and so on. Many IBS sufferers have told us that when they were first diagnosed they had never heard of IBS and they were not given enough information on it. They had no idea it was a common condition and thus felt alone in their complaint.

It seems that many people, apart from coping with the stresses of a chronic illness, have to cope also with GPs who are unsympathetic, disbelieving of their symptoms and dismissive. In some cases the patients are frightened to go back. IBS is not life-threatening and is not a 'serious' illness, but doctors should not underestimate the distress it causes to patients and their families. If you have an unsympathetic doctor, try to make him or her realize how distressing the syndrome is. Perhaps you could encourage him or her to read this book!

Chapter 3

Treating the Problem

'I have tried everything – all sorts of different diets, relaxation tapes, yoga, meditation. I rest as much as possible, try not to get wound up about things. I still work, but I don't strive so hard. I now have a balanced diet, full of fresh fruit and vegetables. I take garlic pills, vitamin pills, evening primrose oil, and a variety of things like that. I'm better than I was, so maybe some of these things do help. I don't know what's contributed to the improvement, so I take all these things just in case!'

In this chapter we are going to discuss the various treatments you may be offered, both by traditional medical practitioners and by alternative ones.

Trying the treatments

The people we spoke to in our research for this book had tried many different ways of helping themselves to cope with IBS. Most people had attacked the problem on many fronts – they had altered their diets and lifestyle in order to find a way of life which minimized their symptoms.

With regard to diets, it is obvious that no one diet suits everyone. Some respondents had found high-fibre diets to be beneficial, others had found low-fibre diets to work best. Others found their symptoms were not so bad when they ate a high-protein/low-fat diet. Some ate very restricted diets, although they were not sure whether these diets were actually helping their symptoms. Most members, however, were trying to ensure a healthy, balanced diet, with plenty of fruit and vegetables and as little junk food as possible.

Along with diet, most members of the Network had tried to alter their lifestyle by trying to live more simply and less stressfully: many had cut down commitments to a minimum, and spent more time relaxing. They tried to act non-competitively at work or in sports, and instead took up walking, relaxation, meditation, yoga and so on and endeavoured to keep calm in the face of stresses. Members also tried a wide range of both traditional and alternative treatments – most trying one treatment after another, hoping they would finally find a 'cure'. These included aromatherapy, homeopathy, acupuncture, hydrotherapy, stress counselling, massage, faith healing and so on. Some members said these had been helpful, other members did not find them so. There was no one treatment that stood out as being more helpful than the rest.

One in twenty of our respondents had such severe pain that they were unable to work and some were on invalidity benefit. Two people could not walk without the aid of a stick, due to severe pain. Others could not perform most of the routine tasks other people take for granted, like cooking, shopping, housework and going on journeys, although luckily this was only a minority of our sample. For all of us, our quality of life is reduced drastically when we first have IBS.

Like the people we spoke to, you will probably find that the medical treatment you are offered is inadequate. However, this is to be expected, since no medication helps all the symptoms of IBS. When asked whether their GPs gave them all the help they could, just over half of our respondents said yes; some qualified their answers by saying that GPs are overworked, or that the treatment and knowledge of IBS is inadequate.

Since we do not yet know what causes IBS, it is difficult to find a treatment that is lastingly effective, or even treatments that would successfully alleviate some of the worst symptoms. It may be that IBS comprises different sorts of disorders, so that what helps one person's symptoms will not help another. However, there are standard treatments which most doctors seem to recommend: these include the prescription of anti-spasmodic drugs to reduce the spasms of the colon and a bulk filler, which helps constipation and diarrhoea by normalizing the stools. Other drugs such as tranquillizers, anti-depressants and painkillers are also prescribed. In addition to being given drugs, over half of all IBS sufferers are advised to go on a high-fibre diet.

As IBS is so common within our society, the cost to the health service is considerable – and, as we shall see, it is debatable whether these treatments have any real effect.

Treating abdominal pain

Some researchers propose that the smooth muscles of the gut are more reactive in IBS sufferers than other people.[1] These muscles can react to various 'triggers', e.g. anxiety, depression, food, traumas, drugs, illness etc. This causes abnormal gut motility, which means that contents pass too quickly or too slowly through the system. This in itself can cause pain. Research has shown that the more stress you have, the more your gut will react with disturbed intestinal motility. Researchers at the London Hospital measured pressure in the small intestines and found that noise and stress altered movements in the small bowels, and that IBS patients reacted more than non-IBS people.[2] Therefore, indirectly, stress can contribute to pain. There is a subset of IBS sufferers who suffer from bad pain most days and, according to Dr Mallinson of Lewisham Hospital, these are the hardest patients to treat. The cause of such chronic pain is unknown. It seems that apart from reducing stress and trying to work through one's emotional problem, there is no lasting cure for chronic pain – a depressing thought. However, some medical treatments may help.

Painkillers
There is a wide range of painkillers on the market, available on prescription or over the counter. From our studies, however, we find that only a fifth of sufferers will be prescribed painkillers, although pain is experienced by most. Nevertheless, other treatments such as anti-spasmodic drugs and anti-diarrhoeal treatments, if they work, can be expected to reduce pain. Aspirin

and paracetamol are painkillers that are generally bought over the counter. Some people take them constantly, which can be harmful. Codeine phosphate, a painkiller which doctors tended to prescribe to our respondents, is a weak narcotic analgesic (painkiller inducing drowsiness). It has a constipating effect – which can be a useful side-effect if you suffer from diarrhoea! Addiction is very unusual, but tolerance does develop (that is to say the effect becomes weaker the more they are taken), so it is better to keep codeine phosphate as an emergency measure.

Some people find the side-effects of strong painkillers distressing enough to discontinue the treatment. One woman, describing why she did not continue with the painkillers, wrote:

'The side effects of the tablets included feeling unwell, dry mouth – a worse feeling than having the pain and anyway they did not help the pain at all.'

Most people who talked about painkillers said that they kept a stock of them, but tried to use them sparingly.

Trying to gain control over the pain by methods other than drugs is covered in Chapter 5.

Anti-spasmodic drugs

Some people find their pain becomes worse after mealtimes, i.e. food is a 'trigger'. However, others find food has no noticeable effect on their IBS symptoms. GPs generally prescribe an anti-spasmodic drug such as Colofac. These work directly on the smooth muscle of the colon to reduce the contractions. Peppermint oil also has a similar effect.

There are two types of anti-spasmodic drugs, those with anti-cholinergic effects and those without. Anti-cholinergic drugs inhibit the motor activity of the stomach, small bowel, and colon. Anti-cholinergic anti-spasmodics such as Merbentyl may be prescribed, but these are unlikely to be the first choice as such drugs have undesirable side-effects such as dry mouth, restlessness, feelings of being 'spaced out', etc. Also, it seems there is little evidence that they actually benefit patients with IBS. Drugs such as Colofac (which do not have anti-cholinergic effects) have been shown to be effective in reducing pain.

Anti-spasmodics may help with the pain, but they have little effect on other symptoms.

'The anti-spasmodic tablets helped a little, but I still knew that it was my own mind that could cure it and not tablets. I am trying to keep off any kind of treatment as I do not wish to be on tablets for the rest of my life, but if I'm bad one day I will take an anti-spasmodic tablet, which aids me a little. I realize I have got to control my feelings.' (Woman, aged 23.)

'I take one sachet of Regulan (bulk filler), two or three Spasmonal capsules (anti-spasmodic) and 1 Colpermin (peppermint) capsule a day. The treatment does not completely eliminate or alleviate the problems of IBS. I still have frequent pain, discomfort and feel very unwell.' (Woman, aged 53.)

Most people did not feel that on its own, anti-spasmodic medication helped them a great deal. This ties in with scientific studies showing that combined treatment (e.g. anti-spasmodic, bulk filler, tranquillizer) gives better results than any one medication alone. It is interesting that although anti-spasmodic drugs are by far the most commonly prescribed drug many sufferers seem to try to control their symptoms without the drugs, and prefer to resort to them when the symptoms are especially bad.

Treatments to reduce wind

Some pain can be due to flatulence. Indeed, if you have had a barium enema you know that when the bowel is filled with air this can re-create some of the pain of IBS. When wind cannot escape from the bowel it causes the bowel to stretch, and this will be felt as a sharp pain.

Why do IBS patients have a problem with wind? One researcher says that excessive gas production associated with carbohydrate intolerance can occur and contributes to symptoms in certain individuals.[3] Carbohydrates and sugars cannot be digested in the small bowel and so they pass into the colon where they are readily fermented, yielding hydrogen and carbon dioxide (gas). Just in case this applies to you, try cutting down the amount of sugars you consume in drinks, cakes, biscuits, sweets etc. However, the main culprit here could be wheat products. Cutting out wheat in the diet is fairly difficult to do, but worth a try. Rice products are a good substitute for wheat.

Lactose deficiency (which will lead to dairy products causing your problems) occurs in five per cent of adults, but the prevalence of lactose malabsorption in IBS patients is not significantly different from that found in other people. There are various home remedies that people have experimented with, including peppermint tea and fennel tea – again, anything is probably worth a try. If you ask your GP to prescribe something for flatulence he or she may suggest peppermint oil. This comes in small capsules and can be bought without prescription at most health shops. Cinnamon, cloves and ginger also help bring up gas. Thompson warns that heartburn is sometimes worsened by taking peppermint.[4]. One of our GPs suggested some yoga positions and exercises; this was also put forward in a book by Shirley Trickett.[5] Charcoal biscuits and pills are supposed to prevent wind: these can be bought at health food shops and some chemists. Charcoal biscuits will make you worse, however, if you are intolerant of wheat products.

Thompson, in his book *Gut Reactions*, devotes a whole chapter to 'burbulence' – wind, belching, gurgling and farting. He explains how these phenomena occur, and how we can help ourselves become less burbulent. For instance, he recommends leaving out fizzy drinks, soufflés and whipped desserts – anything to reduce swallowing air. Don't chew gum, smoke, or talk too much when you are eating. Try to minimize the gastric trapping of air. Avoid foods which lead to flatulence, such as beans. A high-fibre diet may make flatulence worse.

Some patients report that wind is their most difficult symptom:

'The main symptom is wind. I do get a lot of pain, but the wind is not only painful, it's embarrassing. In shops and in other people's houses I frequently have to go to the toilet or go outside. In public, where sometimes I haven't been able to help myself, I see people looking at me as if I'm disgusting. But I can't help it. I just can't. And the doctors can't seem to do anything for wind. They think I'm over-exaggerating it, that I'm neurotic. After all, wind isn't life-threatening – when people have cancer and road accidents a bit of wind? But they don't have to live with it day after d

Treatment for diarrhoea

As described in Chapter 1, diarrhoea can be considered as stools of loose or watery consistency that are passed more frequently than is the individual's normal bowel habit. Diarrhoea is often extremely painful and restricts the sufferer's life considerably. Having to order life around the toilet is extremely difficult, and the difficulty is compounded by the embarrassment felt. There are of course prescribed medicines for diarrhoea but, as with all medicines, they can have side-effects and the long-term efficacy of these drugs is not proven. They are probably best kept for emergencies. Codeine phosphate and loperamide are perhaps the best-known drugs prescribed for the relief of diarrhoea. (Codeine is a painkiller with a constipating effect, hence the prescription for diarrhoea.) However, some of our respondents said that these drugs led to nausea. Both of these drugs reduce gut motility, acting on the smooth muscles of the gut wall. They slow transit time, which means that matter takes longer to pass through the system. Codeine works centrally; this means that as well as acting directly on the gut, it also has effects on the brain. The adverse effects of this drug includes drowsiness, and it should not be taken with tranquillizers or sedatives. Nor should it be taken for long periods of time. Loperamide (Imodium) can be bought over the counter, as its effect is peripheral; this means that it does not affect the brain, but works directly on the gut. If your problem is an alternation of diarrhoea and constipation, then anti-diarrhoeal preparations could cause you to become constipated. Obviously it is better to avoid drugs in cases such as these.

'Between 1978 and 1988 with Merbentyl (anti-spasmodic) and Diconal (painkiller) I coped well, and the diarrhoea completely stopped. My medication was then completely changed to Regulan (bulk filler) and paracetamol and the diarrhoea returned, more severely than in the early days. It has continued for three years. I am now taking eight paracetamol, two Amitryptiline (tranquillizer) and one diactyl tablet every day, but there is no improvement.' (*Woman, aged* 67.)

Presumably this patient's GP decided to take her off Merbentyl because of the anti-cholinergic effects, and off Diconal because it is an opiate. The effects of being on such drugs for over 10 years – i.e. their side-effects and the risk of tolerance – were probably thought to be counter-productive. Although drugs may help in the short-term, we need more innocuous ways of curing ourselves.

'I've got all the drugs, but I try not to take them. However, they're there if I need them. I don't like the effects of some, but I keep the anti-diarrhoeal tablets with me at all times. They always work.'

'I carry an anti-diarrhoeal drug wherever I go. I always feel safe with them, because they work like a dream.'

'I eat arrowroot thickened with juice – I read about it somewhere. It's really helped my diarrhoea.'

If you suffer from diarrhoea, consider whether you want to ask for an anti-diarrhoeal drug. Many of our respondents say they do not like taking drugs; well, this is understandable, but many people find that once they know they can take the tablets if they need to, they no longer need them!

Many people have regular bowel habits, learned when they were young. Those of us with IBS find that our bowel habits become uncontrollable, and this sense of lack of control is one of the worst things about IBS. Professor Read found that 28 per cent of IBS patients in one of his studies had the symptom of 'urgency' and at least 10 per cent of people suffer from bowel incontinence.[6] Such sufferers, Professor Read says, are usually women and their anal sphincter has already been weakened by childbirth. Suddenly having to dash to the toilet, and having an accident if you don't make it, is one of the worst symptoms of IBS, being extremely distressing and embarrassing.

It has been said that we need to retrain our bowels to work more regularly, although this is easier said than done. A psychologist once stated she had trained herself to go to the toilet less often by 'holding on'. This is also given a mention in the Shirley Trickett book. According to a gastroenterologist we consulted, it could not do IBS patients any harm to try to train the bowels in this way.

Treatment for constipation

As described in Chapter 1, constipation can be considered as prolonged gaps between evacuations, and hard stools passed with difficulty. However, everyone has their own individual pattern of bowel movements: some people go once a day, others only three times a week. Constipation will be felt as abdominal discomfort or severe pain.

There are many remedies for constipation, prescribed and non-prescribed. Not all work in the same way – for instance, there are bulking agents, lubricants, chemical stimulants and osmotic laxatives. Some remedies can actually make your IBS worse. The regular use of laxatives can irritate the intestine, and eventually it will not work properly without them. Using laxatives may also put you on the diarrhoea/constipation see-saw. Far safer than laxatives are bulking agents, which may be recommended by your GP for both constipation and diarrhoea. Bulking agents coat the hard faeces, easing their passage through the gut. When taken with fluid they swell up and bulk out the faeces, so that the muscles of the colon expel them from the system more rapidly. Preparations such as Fybogel are made from psyllium, gluten-free dietary fibre. Many GPs recommend a bulking agent as part of a total programme of treatment. However, IBS sufferers must find the correct dose for themselves.

Very few of our respondents said they took laxatives. People who suffered from constipation tended to try to remedy it by eating high-fibre diets, taking bulk fillers and drinking plenty of fluids. According to research, around 20 million laxatives are sold each year; about one in five of the population take laxatives, but many people keep quiet about their need for them. The Eating Disorders Association are anxious that people do not abuse laxatives.[7] They say that such abuse causes dehydration, which can have serious effects on the body – for instance, it can damage vital organs like the kidneys. What is more relevant to IBS sufferers, however, is that laxative abuse can cause permanent damage to the bowel, and prolonged use of laxatives has been linked with bowel tumours. The Eating Disorders Association conducted a survey of their members. Nearly three-quarters had abused, or were currently abusing, laxatives. Their survey revealed many side-effects of laxative abuse including nausca, diarrhoea, constipation, flatulence and digestive difficulties. There were cases of IBS and anal bleeding which members felt were brought on by or exacerbated by laxative abuse. As the undesirable effects of laxatives become more known, hopefully laxative use and abuse will decrease.

For constipation, quite a few of our members recommended eating linseed:

'You sprinkle it on cereal or on yoghurt. You can just swallow it. It doesn't help with the pain but it does help with the constipation. You're supposed to eat one tablespoon three times a day, but I find once a day is enough – it works gently, not like laxatives. This is the only thing I find that works, and I tried everything.'

'You buy it from a health shop. It certainly helps with the constipation, it makes you go naturally – not like some laxatives you can get.'

Tranquillizers and anti-depressants

Tranquillizers are relaxants: they sedate you during the day and make you sleepy at night. The tranquillizers you will be prescribed are likely to be the minor ones.

Barbiturates were the earliest tranquillizers, but these have largely been replaced by the benzodiazepines, of which you probably recognize some of the names: Librium, Valium, Mogadon, Ativan, to mention a few. These are the most popular for mild anxiety and related neuroses. Although these drugs are relatively safe (it is extremely difficult to overdose on them) they are still addictive. Withdrawal symptoms can occur if they are stopped suddenly, and if taken with alcohol they can disturb perception and motor function. GPs usually prescribe tranquillizers in very low doses for IBS, so it is to be hoped that they are quite safe.

Anti-depressants were also prescribed to our respondents, since many patients with IBS are depressed, not surprisingly. The drugs you may be prescribed can be either tricyclics or monoamine oxidase inhibitors (MAOIs). These work in different ways. The tricyclics are more likely to be prescribed, as they are considered safer. Both sorts of drug require several weeks before they take effect and there are side-effects, such as constipation, dizziness and a dry mouth. A frequently prescribed tricyclic anti-depressant is Amitryptiline, which produces fewer side-effects than some of the tricyclics but has sedative effects. Again, your GP may prescribe a low dosage of these drugs, and may recommend you take them only at night. Only you can decide whether or not you want to take these drugs. For those patients who want to know the effects of their drugs we provide a glossary of commonly prescribed drugs for IBS so that they can make an informed choice on whether to take them or not.

Many IBS sufferers will not want to take anti-depressants or tranquillizers because this confirms their fear that IBS is 'all in the mind'. Such medication, however, may be useful in the short term if only because they help you cope with the anxiety you are bound to feel with a disorder such as IBS, although they also have a direct relaxing effect on the gut itself. Nevertheless, the worry about dependency and side effects may mean you don't want to risk taking them. Tranquillizers and/or anti-depressants were prescribed to a third of the people we talked to during the course of our research.

It is important that you do not feel pressurized into taking tranquillizers or anti-depressants. Remember you have a choice, and make sure you discuss any reservations you have about your treatments with your doctor.

Various researchers have found that a combined treatment programme works best, i.e. a tranquillizer or anti-depressant, smooth muscle relaxant and a bulking agent.[8] However, not all people who receive this treatment experience a sustained improvement in their symptoms.

'IBS seems to be very complex and I doubt whether two people have the same symptoms. I saw a gastroenterologist who confirmed there's no cure, but I went on holiday equipped with medication from my doctor for diarrhoea and constipation, and between the two thoroughly enjoyed my holiday! I'm not going to let IBS spoil my lifestyle. All one needs is an understanding doctor.'

'I am taking part in a drug trial using sulpiride in small doses (normally used to treat schizophrenics). It helped a bit but I did not receive advice on self-help and other ways of treating and coping with the unpleasant symptoms.'

We should mention that sulpiride, a major tranquillizer, is not normally prescribed.

Psychological treatments

In 1987 a team of researchers evaluated studies which had investigated psychological treatments of IBS.[9] These included psychotherapy, focusing on increasing insight and self-reliance, relaxation, education about IBS and group therapy concentrating on life stresses and problems, hypnotherapy and bowel sound biofeedback (where patients can hear their bowel sounds via an electronic stethoscope). The researchers suggested several treatments should be tried together: they believe sufferers should be educated about the workings of the digestive system and the range of normal bowel functioning; they should be taught progressive muscle relaxation and be given biofeedback and therapy aimed at coping with stress. The researchers found that most of their patients improved on this treatment and concluded that psychological treatments should be either more intensive or more comprehensive to deal adequately with a large proportion of the IBS population. Such treatment, however, is unlikely to be available generally on the NHS because of the enormous cost.

Psychotherapy
Obviously psychotherapy will help some patients more than others, and even some symptoms are more responsive than others: another team of researchers who studied 102 IBS patients found that psychotherapy worked best with symptoms such as diarrhoea and intermittent abdominal pain.[10] Patients were either given medical treatment alone (anti-spasmodic drug and a bulking agent) or medical treatment plus seven sessions of psychotherapy. The psychotherapy group were also given a relaxation tape to use on a regular basis at home.

The researchers found that on examination after treatment, and again six months later, the patients who were in the psychotherapy group had improved more than those who had been given medication only. Psychotherapy was not as much help for patients with constipation and constant pain. People with emotional problems were improved in their symptoms, probably due to a reduction of anxiety or depression after the therapy. The team say that this may be because anxiety and/or depression causes bowel dysfunction in at least some patients with IBS. But there are other explanations and however IBS is caused, living with such a chronic condition can itself lead to psychological problems. People with IBS are, not surprisingly, more depressed and anxious than healthy people. Some people believe that IBS is the result of depression and anxiety, while others hold that the depression and anxiety is a result of having a disorder which nobody seems to know how to cure and which is not taken as seriously as it should be. However, if psychotherapy helps sufferers feel better it doesn't much matter which of these is true.

According to Peter Whorwell, psychotherapy is beneficial and is worth considering. [11] If you can get psychological treatment on the NHS, go ahead and have a go!

Carol is a professional woman in her mid-thirties:

'I have been seeing Dr F. on a six-weekly basis for about a year now. I was referred to Dr F. by the gastroenterologist who had exhausted his treatment and that was the only thing we hadn't considered. I was reluctant at first, but on the other hand I felt that I had to try everything. I was so frustrated at the doctors not having found anything tangible that a psychological link would have been better than nothing and would at least have given me something to work on.

'It was explained to me that the purpose of psychotherapy was to see if there was anything emotional that I had buried in the past which was not noticeable when I had a "well" gut but which is now manifesting itself in the form of pain etc. now that I have an "unwell" gut. I can remember my first visit to see Dr F. I had been feeling dreadful all day at work – the pain was so bad that I had been pacing around the office (this is how I feel *every* day). I was worried about how I was going to get through my meeting with Dr F. because I guessed it would mean my having to sit down for up to an hour, which I would find so uncomfortable. My office friends said that I should ask Dr F. if I could talk to him while lying down, because if anyone should understand how I felt then he should. When I arrived I explained my need to lie down. Dr F.'s reply was to tell me to sit down and see if it got any better. I couldn't seem to get through to him that sitting made it worse and that the way I felt that day was how I feel every day and was not in any way connected with being nervous about our meeting.

'Dr F.'s attitude does not seem to have altered to this day. For example, on my last visit I stood up after about ten minutes and he asked me why I had stood up at that particular moment. In other words, were we talking about something which had touched a raw nerve, thus making my symptoms worse – I could have cheerfully swung for him! Dr F. has discussed with me all areas of my life. One angle he explored was the possibility that my IBS was connected to the fact that I was in my thirties and unmarried! Why wasn't I married? Why wasn't I in a long-term relationship? Where are my children? I'm not normal! I have tried explaining to Dr F. that I believe one shouldn't succumb to the pressure to be married, and one should marry when one feels it's the right thing to do. I believe that a person should not be made to feel abnormal if they choose to remain single. In my opinion, a person can lead a happy and fulfilled life without marriage. Dr F. kept on implying that I had a "problem". I told him that surely it is only a problem if one is unhappy. I'm not unhappy with my life, apart from IBS. I see myself as "sitting on the fence", i.e. a long-term relationship with children with the right person looks inviting but equally dating lots of different men and having lots of fun looks equally good too. It would take someone really special to make me take the leap. How on earth has this got anything to do with IBS?

'I don't think psychotherapy has helped me in any way whatsoever, nor do I think it ever will. The only benefit I could get from it would be to discuss the stresses and strains of having IBS and how I was coping with it. Sometimes I feel guilty about moaning to my friends about my IBS so I tend to keep quiet and let the frustration build up. After all, they heard all this three years ago and to continue moaning about it would just be going over the same old ground. There's nothing more to say, nothing more to add. I feel Dr F. has been patronizing. He hasn't got a clue. This is nothing personal as I am sure he is a kind man and means well, but I don't know how much longer I shall continue trying to explain to Dr F. that the only underlying emotional problem contributing to my IBS is the actual strain of having IBS."

Anne has a totally different story, however. Although reluctant at first to be sent to a psychiatrist, she found that he was the only one who really understood and helped her. When one of us first went to see Anne her IBS symptoms were uncontrollable; she was in a lot of pain and suffered badly with diarrhoea and flatulence.

She had lost a lot of weight, and was struggling to hold down a responsible job. She knew no one with IBS, and did not confide in others about her problems. She was becoming weaker and weaker, and more depressed by the day. Her GP did not seem to be helpful – she felt he dismissed her symptoms and believed she was neurotic. She did not feel she wanted to keep going back to her GP, who never seemed to offer any help. However, eventually he persuaded her to go to a psychiatrist, saying there must be a reason why she 'keeps getting all these symptoms'. Although Anne did not want to go to the psychiatrist, she now feels it's the best thing that happened to her. Anne sees Dr P. regularly, and talks through all her problems and anxieties with him. She is lucky in that Dr P. seems to understand:

'Until four years ago I was fine, went out to parties, travelled everywhere etc. Then I began to get all these symptoms. I went to my GP, who thought I'd imagined it all; he thought IBS wasn't serious and I should just get on with it. He didn't understand, he didn't help. I felt weak, ill, my life was so miserable I just kept going back to him all the time, so in the end he thought I must have something psychologically wrong with me. He insisted I go to a psychiatrist but at first I wouldn't. However, over the course of a couple more visits he kept on about it, and because I didn't have any choice I thought I had better go because I do need help. When I did go I found him helpful. He was understanding, and really listened to me. He takes me seriously, he believes me when I say how bad I feel. I decided I would keep on going to see him because he promised me that if he couldn't help me get better he would send me to a consultant. He's helped me, because he actually believed that IBS is a problem. He believed that how I felt was genuine, and that it wasn't all in my mind. He could see that I was weak, and believed me whereas the GP wouldn't. I could hardly get up the stairs to my GP, and I nearly collapsed one day. The GP acted as if I made it up. Dr P. hasn't got rid of my symptoms, but could see that I couldn't go on, and he made me stop work. He thought I should because I was so ill, and travelling to town each day was making me far worse. Stopping work has helped me in a lot of ways. If I hadn't gone to him, I'm sure I would have had a nervous breakdown. He's been very good to me; if it wasn't for him I don't know what I would have done.'

Hypnotherapy

Leading gastroenterologist Peter Whorwell says that his research group has been looking at the effect of hypnotherapy for several years, and finds that approximately 80 per cent of patients who have been difficult to treat with other methods respond well to it. [12] According to Dr Chris Mallinson of Lewisham Hospital, about eight out of ten patients undergoing hypnotherapy lose their symptoms apparently permanently or certainly for over a year. [13] These are often the patients for whom conventional treatment – tablets, powders and dietary advice – has not worked. Dr Whorwell says that it isn't all in the mind – actual physiological effects can take place, for example the rectal area can become less or more sensitive. [14] This is Sue's account of a visit to Dr Whorwell's clinic in Manchester:

'Dr Whorwell is well-known for his treatment of IBS by using hypnotherapy. His success rate is high, especially with long-term sufferers. Nevertheless, in view of the time-consuming nature of the treatment – it is on a one-to-one basis and each session can last up to half an hour – and lack of sufficient funds, hypnotherapy is seen as a last resort treatment, to be tried when all else fails.

'We were able to sit in on two people being hypnotized. This was extremely interesting as neither of us had seen anything like it before. The hypnotist (Liz) started by talking to each patient about how they had felt since she had last seen them, and whether they were worried about any up and coming events.

'The hypnotherapy itself seemed to me to be like someone talking you through a relaxation exercise. Liz talked each patient into a state of deep relaxation and then concentrated on telling them about the positive ways in which they could control their bowels. She uses soothing imagery to relax and then tells the sufferers about their own strengths and capabilities. She tells them that they are in control of their bowels and their lives, that they will be able to cope with any difficulties during the coming week, that they feel confident and relaxed. Coping with IBS is inextricably linked to coping with life.

'We asked the patients what they thought of the hypnotherapy. They were both enthusiastic. It had helped them a great deal and made them feel more in control.

'The hypnotherapist assured us that hypnotherapy is more than just inducing a state of deep relaxation. From research it is apparent that it will slow down colonic activity, although how this happens is not known. We asked if anyone can be hypnotized and were told that eight out of ten people are able to "go under". We were also assured, as I'd heard before, that the hypnotist doesn't have control over the patient and cannot make her/him do anything she/he would not normally do.'

Here are two of our members' experiences of hypnotherapy:

'I decided to try hypnosis for my IBS with great trepidation. I think to most of us the word hypnosis brings to mind the typical stage act with people being made to do silly or strange things without knowing they are doing them. Believe me, this is not possible. I found a qualified GP who also practised hypnosis as I felt that he would know about IBS and what the range of symptoms includes. I was lucky in that when I first met the doctor he was very pleasant, understanding and "normal". He did not charge me for the first appointment, during which he explained about hypnosis, how it works, how you should feel etc. He also explained that different people can be hypnotized to different levels, for example if you are a relaxed person you are likely to respond more easily than someone who is tense. He then hypnotized me for a short while to let me decide if I wanted to go ahead with treatment. By this time I had got myself into quite a state worrying about what was going to happen to me, so I was very surprised that once I was lying down and he had started to count I could gradually feel myself relaxing and feeling more and more comfortable. I left the surgery wondering what on earth I had been worrying about as I had been pleasantly surprised by how simple it all was and how relaxed I felt.

'I had six appointments and although I did not actually have any improvement in my IBS symptoms during that time I was gradually feeling more relaxed generally. I felt I would have liked more appointments but the doctor said I had progressed as I should and that if I used the cassette he had recorded for me two to three times a week I should see further improvement. He also said that if in the future I felt I wanted to take things further he could attempt to hypnotize me to a deeper state where he could look into my past to see if there was anything there that could have triggered IBS but this could be a very upsetting experience and that it needed careful consideration as to whether some things are best left in the past.

'Within a couple of weeks of finishing the hypnotherapy I did have three months when my IBS was a lot better and I do think it was because I had a time of being more relaxed. The problem I found with being left to use the cassette was finding the right time to listen to it because you need complete privacy and the peace of mind to know you are not going to be disturbed so that you can relax completely. I have not been able to use the cassette regularly as at present I have a four-year-old and very little privacy. When she goes to school I do intend using the cassette regularly and will see if I get any improvement again. The only question mark left for me about hypnosis is whether one hynotherapist's treatment would be different from another's. My hypnotherapist only used relaxation suggestions and I wonder if another one would refer to the IBS and make suggestions to you about ways of controlling the symptoms?

A man in his twenties gives the second account:

'The first thing I do when I go for my hypnotherapy sessions is to answer questionnaires about my symptoms: pain, bloating, diarrhoea and so on. I have to mark on a scale how bad my symptoms have been. Then I talk to her about my week, what I've been doing, whether it was a good or bad week. It's like a mini counselling session. The last was my sixth session (out of ten) and the doctor compares my notes now with my notes from the last session. This is all before the session begins. Then I sit down and close my eyes and relax for the session. She tells me to relax, to think of my abdomen, to hold my hands over my abdomen . . . she keeps telling me to relax, saying this warm feeling over my stomach is taking the pain away. She builds it up over the twenty or so minutes . . . saying the feeling is getting hotter and all the time telling me to relax. Then towards the end of the session she'll say things like, "You will be confident . . . you can take on anything", and so on.

'I feel very relaxed after the sessions. I'm fully aware of everything that's going on around me. I'm quite clear that the reason my symptoms have improved so much is the hypnotherapy. I had all sorts of drugs before, they didn't help me in the slightest, but this is really good. I also have tapes given to me by the doctor which I try to use every day. I'm very lucky, because all this is on the NHS.

Complementary treatments

Evening primrose oil
Workers at Addenbrookes Hospital, Cambridge, conducted a study in which they found that women whose IBS symptoms were severe during their menstrual period were helped by taking evening primrose oil.[15] One group of women took eight Efamol capsules containing 500 mg of evening primrose oil daily, and another group took placebo capsules (containing olive oil). They

found that just over half the patients taking the Efamol reported an improvement in symptoms, while none of those taking the olive oil capsules improved. This seems a strong effect. However, improvement did not take place straight away – it usually began in the second month of administration, but in some cases was not apparent for over three months. The researchers suggest that their IBS patients may be deficient in some essential fatty acids that are contained in evening primrose oil. It is not suggested that evening primrose oil will help all IBS patients – just women whose symptoms seem to vary with the menstrual cycle. Women with IBS should keep a diary of symptoms, and see whether this is the case. If so, they should see their doctor and discuss the possibility of taking evening primrose oil. However, evening primrose oil is very expensive and its benefits are not proven.

Diet

Many sufferers have been told by their GPs to eat a high-fibre diet. However, some sufferers find that this can actually make the problem worse, especially if the fibre is wheat-derived and the problem is mainly diarrhoea. One of us had been on a high-fibre vegetarian diet for fourteen years when IBS symptoms such as occasional abdominal pain and constipation became constant and severe, despite a healthy lifestyle which included plenty of exercise. Constipation changed to diarrhoea, and the high-fibre diet only seemed to make this worse.

What is the evidence on high-fibre diets, and why are doctors still recommending them? McCloy and McCloy state that a report from the Royal College of Physicians failed to establish a link between dietary fibre and gastrointestinal disorders.[16] Also, there seems to be no difference in the amount of fibre taken by IBS and non-IBS people. Bran may not be a good idea for people with IBS as it has other effects on the bowel apart from acting as a bulking agent. It prevents the absorption of calcium and bile, and increases the levels of prostaglandins (chemicals which produce pain). We do not know what effects this has on gut motility, but many IBS sufferers find bran aggravates their symptoms. Researchers suggest that a low-fat, high-protein diet may help instead. Controlling your IBS through diet is discussed in the next chapter.

Homeopathy
Homeopathy was founded by an eighteenth-century physician called Dr Samuel Hahnemann. It is based on the principle that disorders can be treated by giving small quantities of a substance which, in larger doses, would bring on the symptoms that the homeopath is trying to treat. This is often called 'treating like with like'. The quantities given are very small indeed – the substance is distilled and diluted until its final concentration is so small it cannot be measured. Homeopathic medicine is said to stimulate the body's own defences in order to cure the patient. Homeopathy is a holistic practice – that is, the practitioner treats the whole person rather than his or her disorder alone. The first consultation is therefore likely to be a lengthy process whereby the homeopath asks you all sorts of questions about your lifestyle as well as your disorder. This means that the homeopath may give you one remedy and your friend another, although you may both be there for your IBS. Homeopathy is said to have no harmful effects, and many people say they have benefited from it. Further details can be obtained from the British Homeopathic Association (see Appendix II).

Aromatherapy
Aromatherapy treats illness by using essential oils, which may be added to the bath, inhaled or rubbed into the skin. The aromatherapist takes a history of the patient and chooses the most appropriate oils for his or her complaint, also taking into consideration lifestyle and personal habits. Certain oils are thought to help lift depressions, others are thought to combat stress. The oils can be massaged over the body, which is thought to be doubly beneficial as massage is known to release hormones with a calming effect.

Colonic irrigation
This treatment is making a come-back. It is possible to go to a colon clinic and have a bowel wash-out. This is similar to enema – warm water is infused into the large intestine through the anus and flows up, along with accumulated matter. Cleansing the colon, whether by enemas, irrigation or purgatives (strong

laxatives) has been said to be beneficial throughout the ages. However, whether colonic irrigation does have any discernible benefits is open to discussion; Dr Mallinson's view is that any benefits are strictly short-term.[17] Professor Read says that colonic irrigation can provide temporary relief, but it is certainly not a long-term cure.[18]

Faith healing

Healing by the laying-on of hands is generally performed free or at little cost as such healing is often part of the healer's service to the community, inspired by religious beliefs. Often you give a donation, as large or small as you want. Spiritual healers tend to believe that there is a flow of energy from a higher force, or God, which can heal through the medium of the healer. It is often said that disbelievers can 'block' the healing energy by setting up a 'barrier'.

'In 1984 I had ten sessions with a lady healer which I'm convinced did a lot of good. Since then the pains have been very infrequent and of much less severity.' (*Man aged sixty-seven.*)

'I went to a spiritualist place. I sat in a warm room and the woman put relaxing music on – it was very nice. Then she put her hands on my shoulders and asked me if I felt the warmth. She said it was energy flowing through her to me, as a vessel of God. I did feel a warmth, but I believed it was just the pressure of her hands. She then moved her hands around various parts of my body. I didn't like it, I felt uncomfortable, and what's more I couldn't believe in it. I wanted to, but I couldn't. I went about six times but I never felt any different; she said it was because I was resisting belief.'

Naturopathy

Naturopathy believe that people have become ill because they have moved away from a 'natural' lifestyle: our eating and drinking habits, work and exercise patterns are far removed from the simple, natural lives people led when they were hunter-gatherers. Consequently a naturopath prescribes treatment based on a simple, natural way of life which includes fasting and special diets such as a natural wholefood diet without additives, a macrobiotic diet or a rice diet. The diets are generally low in sugar and salt, and include plenty of fresh fruit and vegetables. Naturopaths often recommend vitamin and mineral supplements, and exercise and relaxation techniques to deal with stress.

Acupuncture

Acupuncture is one of the oldest forms of treatment, originating in China. The acupuncturist stimulates points on the surface of the body by inserting sterile needles in specific places. The needles are either left untouched for 15–20 minutes or moved up and down in order to stimulate the 'channels of energy'. Acupuncturists believe that illness results when the body is in a state of imbalance; when the biological and emotional functions are upset, the energy does not flow properly through the invisible energy lines throughout the body. Acupuncturists seek to restore the balance by stimulating the specific points along the energy channels.

Some people find acupuncture very helpful, as illustrated by one of our respondents:

'I have two very accurate indicators of the degree of stress in my life. Both I could do without! One is eczema on my hands and the other is IBS. My IBS began even as a toddler. As a child I sat for hours at the bottom of the stairs, hugging my tummy before heading off for school. As my life went on I learnt to accept that I would have to rush to the toilet five, six or even seven times before an appointment, and that exams would be accompanied by severe gut ache. No one seemed to question it so I thought that I'd go on like that for ever.

'In my first job after university I found myself under a great deal of pressure and at the same time my personal life was going badly wrong. My IBS took over with a vengeance and become the centre of my life for some months. I was being sick, spending large chunks of time rushing to the toilet and generally feeling wretched. Doctors and hospital appointments left me feeling more hopeless. I was given anti-spasmodic tablets and left with the assumption that this would be it for the rest of my life – not a very attractive prospect.

'At that time acupuncture was pretty new on the British health scene and a friend and I wondered if it could help us over hay fever. Never thinking that it could help my problems with my gut, I went off to my first appointment. When the acupuncturist put the first needle in my hand to show me that it didn't hurt, my hand become red and throbbed. Puzzled, I told him that although it wasn't hurting, it certainly was doing something.

'The acupuncturist asked if I had something wrong with my large intestine. When I told him my history he said that he could probably cure that but not to hold out great hope for my hay fever. I could have kissed him!

'Six treatments later, I felt well enough to take some decision about my life which started to relieve some of the stress I was under. Up until that time, I felt so terrible that I couldn't see a way forward at all. After eight treatments I was able to stop going to the acupuncturist with the knowledge that I could go back if I needed to.

'That was sixteen years ago. I am still someone whom stress first strikes in the gut, the difference is that I feel that I can do something about it. When my gut gets bad I make an appointment to see the acupuncturist, have a few treatments and I'm back to normal. In fact, there haven't been so many times since that first lot of treatment that I have got that bad. I feel that knowing that there is something that will relieve the symptoms is part of the battle and helps me to keep my guts under control.'

However, two other members, both women in their thirties, found the experience unpleasant:

'After trying acupuncture, the practitioner said she didn't know what else to do. I found acupuncture extremely uncomfortable and sometimes painful and was relieved to give it up.'

'I only went four times. The woman put needles in my stomach, but mostly in my legs. They tingled but were not particularly painful. Then she left the room for twenty minutes. During this time the needles became more and more painful. I wanted to pull them out but was scared in case I pulled them out wrongly or something. I didn't like to call out – I didn't know whereabouts in the building she was. So I waited. When she came back I told her to get the needles out quickly it was so painful. She said I should have called out. It didn't improve my symptoms at all – if anything, it made them worse. The woman said the pains were due to my negativity. I never went back.'

Meditation

Meditation for health and harmony has been used for thousands of years, and there are now many forms of meditation. Basically, though, meditation involves sitting comfortably in a quiet place, and focusing your mind – either through looking at a selected object, like a candle, or repeating one word for the duration of the meditation. The word is called a 'mantra'. Concentrating on the one word, or on your breathing, can help focus attention and calm the mind. When somebody meditates, his or her breathing slows down, as does the heart rate. Meditation relaxes the muscles, and reduces oxygen consumption. When you practise meditation regularly, you may find that you can respond much more calmly to stressful situations.

Although you can meditate without learning the technique from others, or from books, you will find it easier to meditate if you obtain some simple books on meditation – these should be available from your local library. There are courses teaching meditation – for instance, a popular one is transcendental meditation (TM) – associated with the sixties and the Beatles. This involves sitting with your eyes closed for twenty minutes twice a day, repeating a mantra. The mantra is chosen for you by a teacher of TM to suit your particular personality. The word is meant to be as relaxing and tranquillizing as possible.

Meditation is said to relieve tiredness, dissolve deep-rooted stress and leave the system feeling calmer and more alert. Some IBS sufferers have found meditation very helpful.

Relaxation
The few books that are written for the IBS sufferer all recommend relaxation as a way of coping with IBS. This is not surprising, as any pain or medical complaint is aggravated by worrying, tension and stress. It is well known that people with the same complaint will experience pain differently; people who try to maintain a positive outlook, however hard this is, fare better than those who become depressed and believe that they will never recover. [19] Consequently, any technique that decreases your stress levels and helps you to take life at a more even pace must be beneficial.

One of the best ways to relax is to learn to breathe properly. Many of us breathe too shallowly at the best of times and, in times of tension or pain, almost forget to breathe at all! Your body needs a good supply of oxygen at such times and deep breathing will help you to calm down.

Try this simple exercise for about ten minutes:

Sit on a straight-backed chair with your feet flat on the floor (if your legs are too short, put a cushion under your feet). Keep your spine straight – imagine a thread attached to the crown of your head pulling it up towards the ceiling. Rest your hands loosely in your lap.

Breathe slowly and deeply through your nose. Concentrate on the rise and fall of your navel. As you breathe in say to yourself 'peace in' and as you breathe out, say 'tension out'. Imagine the good, peaceful feelings that you are breathing in and all the worry, stress and bad feeling that you are breathing out.

You may also like to try this calming exercise:

Stand with your feet hip-distance apart with your arms loosely by your sides. As you breathe in, slowly raise your arms out to the sides and up above your head. Hold the breath and stretch as far as you can with your arms. Then slowly exhale and lower your arms. Repeat, to the rhythm of your breathing, six times at first, increasing as you practise more. If the arm movements are done slowly it will encourage you to breathe in and out more deeply.

The following exercise is often used by teachers of yoga and other relaxation methods to relax the whole body:

In a warm, quiet room where you won't be disturbed, lie on your back on the floor or sit in a straight-backed chair. Rest your arms by your sides if you are lying down, or loosely in your lap if you are sitting, with the palms uppermost. Concentrate on breathing deeply and slowly, feeling the gentle rise and fall movement of your navel.

Imagine your feet and tense each one by pointing it downwards and curling your toes, and then relaxing. Tense your lower leg by pointing your foot towards your head, feeling the stretch, then relax and repeat on the other side. Tense and relax your knees and your thighs. Move up to your buttocks and then your stomach and tense, then relax the muscles there. Think of the small of your back, tense and then relax it. Move up your back and think about tensing then relaxing your shoulders and your chest. Clench your fist tightly and then relax and let go. Repeat with the other hand. Tense and then relax your upper and lower arms. Move up to your neck, tense and relax the muscles there. Tense your jaw and chin, then relax them. Clench your teeth together and pull your mouth into a big, false smile, then relax. Close your eyes tightly and wrinkle up your nose, then release the tension. Raise your eyebrows as high as you can and relax them. Go through all the parts of your body, thinking about tensing then relaxing them. Be aware of how the muscles feel when they are tense and how they feel after you relax them.

Continuing to breathe slowly and deeply, let your body give up to the pull of gravity. Rest like this for at least ten minutes. Concentrate on your breathing. If any unwanted thoughts come to mind, let them come up and through you and out of you.

As you complete the relaxation, begin to move your feet and legs, then your hands and arms. Move your neck and head and slowly open your eyes.

If you find relaxation helpful you will probably want to take it further. Shirley Trickett has a chapter on deep relaxation, and shows you how to practise this technique.[20] You can also buy relaxation tapes in chemists and health shops.

The whole treatment

Looking at all the data from our questionnaires, it is obvious that most people use the medication they are prescribed some of the time. Sufferers feel unhappy because they cannot find relief from all, or even most, of their symptoms. (All sufferers suffer from several symptoms, of course; this is what qualifies IBS as a syndrome.) However, sufferers could generally find some medication to take which helped on occasions, and even this is better than nothing. Pain was obviously the most difficult symptom to treat.

To sum up, you really do need to attack the IBS problem from all directions: try different diets, different medications, keep yourself healthy by eating nutritious food and make sure you get enough rest. If alternative medicine appeals to you, then perhaps you should try that. However, some people have spent vast amounts of money trying to cure themselves, only to find the symptoms persist; you have to weigh up the advantages of trying such treatments against the costs. However hard it is (and it is hard!), try to maintain a positive outlook and make sure your GP understands the problems IBS can cause as a good doctor can be a source of strength.

Chapter 4

Physical and Psychological Consequences

'I live from hour to hour and avoid making plans in advance. IBS has changed my life – I work, travel and so on around my symptoms.'

Living with IBS can mean a very restricted life. It may prevent you doing things other people take for granted – for instance shopping, car and bus journeys, long-distance travel, going for walks or visiting friends. It may prevent you from doing the sort of work you'd like to do, or even working at all.

If diarrhoea is a problem you may find yourself having to plan around the availability of toilets in everything you do; if pain is one of your symptoms you may be stopped from doing things because the agony keeps you at home in bed; if you are constipated you may find you have to keep to a specific routine; if you suffer from wind you may only want to see people in the open air, or not at all. Women with bloating sometimes have to put up with people asking them when their baby is due! Some of the symptoms of IBS can be a great embarrassment: – wind, incontinence, having to rush to the toilet, being doubled up with pain – these alone can prevent sufferers from socializing. Isolation and depression can follow.

Many IBS sufferers will tell of the psychological effects of having to live with the condition. It may be hard to cope with for a number of reasons. IBS lacks validity and a sufferer may find that doctors and family are far from understanding and sympathetic. It seems to be the luck of the draw whether you get support and useful information from your GP or from gastroenterologists, although specialists with a particular interest in IBS, and their staff, can be more sympathetic. At the moment, the medical profession has little to offer in the way of effective treatment. 'There are no known clinical tests that will confirm or refute the diagnosis with certainty and there is no specific therapy for the condition,' say researchers on a study into IBS.[1] Although medical professionals are advocating that IBS is diagnosed on a positive basis, i.e. on the basis of the presence of particular symptoms, it is still, in practice, a diagnosis of exclusion – in other words, it's what you've got if you haven't got anything else! You may go through a series of uncomfortable or painful tests only to be told there's nothing wrong with you, try a high fibre diet/take these anti-spasmodics/this bulking agent, and there's not much else that can be done to help you. You may be given tranquillizers or anti-depressants and told to reduce the stress in your life, but as Louise, a 32-year-old housewife, says, 'It's having to live with IBS that causes me the most stress.'

Family and friends may not understand and you may feel they see you as lazy or wanting attention, or being unable to cope with life. Because of the attitudes of others, and sometimes of the medical profession, it is not uncommon for IBS sufferers to blame themselves or feel guilty about their condition. However, a supportive GP, relative or friend can make all the difference.

The symptoms themselves are hard to cope with. Quite apart from the main symptoms of diarrhoea and/or constipation, abdominal pain, bloating and wind, there may be secondary symptoms. For instance, many people with IBS experience panic attacks – a racing heart, difficulty in breathing, sweating, a feeling of faintness and sickness. This can be a very frightening experience that can make you think twice about putting yourself in the same situation again. The panic attack may be caused by the fact that you were in a place where no toilet was nearby and you feared you were going to have an accident. Indeed, you may not have made it to the toilet in time – incontinence is more common than people realize. Thereafter, that location – whether it was in a supermarket, on the street, or even at home – can bring on feelings of panic because you fear it happening again. Consequently you avoid those situations, or suffer great anxiety when you are forced into them.

Sufferers may develop obsessions or other behaviour that seems strange to non-sufferers. You may feel safer or more comfortable in certain clothes, you may take to wearing incontinence pads or sanitary towels, you may not be able to leave the house without going to the toilet many times, you may not be able to eat in public, you may not feel able to stay at friends' homes, you may have to avoid morning appointments or events in the evening, you may develop routines in the morning or at bedtime that cannot be broken without causing you anxiety. These limitations will be understandable to other IBS sufferers, but you may not feel able to explain why you can't go out for a meal with a friend or for a drink with work colleagues, for example. Therefore, you may resort to elaborate behaviour patterns. You make bizarre excuses to avoid situations that make you anxious: you'd rather be thought to be unfriendly or unsociable than explain why you can't go out for a meal; you go out of your way to avoid someone you know in the street in case she stops to talk and you want to go to the toilet, or are in pain, or need to fart . . .

Needless to say, the person with IBS can become isolated and depressed and may feel ashamed of their behaviour, or inadequate about their inability to cope. But coping is just what you are doing – coping in the ways that are available to you. (see Chapter 5 for more on coping).

When sufferers do not feel they cope well with their IBS, depression can be the result.

'I cope very badly. I'm in tears most days as it's so bad when I get up and continues through the day and night. I get very frightened of going to work and sitting all day with so much congestion and pain, with nowhere to go to alleviate it,' *says Sheila.*

Some people have sought psychiatric treatment because of the stress and anxiety they suffer. Many do not feel optimistic that their IBS will improve, especially if they've had it some time and it hasn't got better, or has even got worse.

Other secondary symptoms include fatigue and lethargy, when you are unable to do anything but curl up with a hot-water bottle. This adds to the frustration, you feel that your life is passing you by. There are so many things you want to do, but are prevented from doing.

'I feel that four years out of the five I've had IBS have been ruined, wasted,' *says Pat, a thirty-seven-year-old secretary.*

'I don't have any leisure activities at all. I gave them all up. For four years I didn't go anywhere on holiday, or go to a restaurant; I didn't eat in the street in case I couldn't find a loo, I didn't visit anyone, and I stood at the back of the church where the loo was. In the cinema I have to sit in the end seat, in case.'

Many sufferers worry about the future. How will they cope with their IBS? What jobs will they be able to do? They worry about having panic attacks, about incontinence and pain, about not being in control of their own body.

Why is it so common to find that people with IBS feel somehow it is their fault, and why does guilt often accompany an attack?

'I get so depressed and fed up with myself because it's not fair on my son to find me in bed all the time when he gets home from school,' *says Becky, a single parent with a twelve year-old son.*

'I always felt like a hypochondriac so played down my symptoms at consultations.'

'The doctors were pleasant but made me feel inadequate because I couldn't cope with IBS.'

'I would probably have felt too guilty at being stupid enough to have IBS to join a self-help group. I always feel I should cope better.'

Again, it is usually the attitudes of people, who don't have IBS that make us feel this way.

'I'm fed up with being told, however indirectly, that I'm some kind of stressed-up failure who likes to be the way I am because I either want to avoid life or am lazy!'

'I am fed up with having a reputation for being late or thought of as being lazy. It is impossible to explain to someone who is 'normal' how you can have been up since before 7 am but still find it difficult to get out by 9 am.'

Embarrassment is common. Bowels and their problems are, at best, an unglamorous subject. Some people find having IBS more embarrassing than others. Claudia describes how she feels:

'I would die if anyone knew about it. To even my closest friends this is top secret and I spend my life inventing excuses for why I can't do things. The distressing thing is that I would love to join in and do things other people do, but my life depends on my stomach.'

Claudia has had IBS since she was sixteen. She is now forty-two. She was only diagnosed three years ago and during the previous twenty-three years she presumed she was a 'nervous wreck'.

'When I was eventually referred to a specialist I was quite relieved that it was a recognized problem. Perhaps someone somewhere had had it before!'

She goes on to describe how it all began:

'We moved south when I was sixteen. I joined the sixth form down here and then the problems started. I had to leave school after three months of hell, much to my parents' disappointment. Like them, I too expected I would go on to university and get a good job, but now I couldn't even sit in a classroom for thirty minutes. Even sitting in the doctor's waiting room was a trial. No one understood. I began to feel I was mental and made up all sorts of reasons about having to leave school to look after my sick mother. I was taken to see psychiatrists and diagnosed as having 'nerve problems'.

'When I was a teenager I think I was regarded as a freak as I always wanted the TV or radio on to drown my stomach. I am still the same now but, being a housewife, at least I am in charge of the situation at home. The problems start at other people's houses. People began to think I had a fear of 'quiet' so I had to let them think that. It was less embarrassing. Saying you are claustrophobic gets you a seat on the end of the row in a theatre or restaurant so that you can dash to the loo. Having a migraine is useful for getting out of things you just can't face.

'I now have three children and they have been marvellous to hide behind. You can always leave anywhere to take a child to the loo (and go yourself) and you can always talk and make noises with a child in a quiet situation, for example doctors' and dentists' waiting rooms.

'I find it impossible to attend talks at the children's schools. I dread parents' evenings. In fact, I don't eat for three days beforehand in case that will help. I dread things months ahead because I don't know how I can get out of them.

I can't go to church because I can't sit throught the sermon. They asked me to be a school governor but I had to leave the meeting to go to the loo so I made excuses to get out of that. People think I'm afraid of commitment – but it's not that.

'All in all, to everyone else, I am a likeable person, but because of all these problems they probably think I am a bag of nerves. I am not. All I need is a new stomach.'

Having IBS in this society can, as Claudia describes, seriously influence a person's behaviour. Dora, who has had it for fourteen years, writes about the lasting effects on her:

'After all these years the actual bouts of IBS are rare and short-lived but unfortunately, what is almost worse, I have been left with a terrible phobia about being in any situation where I do not have easy access to a toilet. The panic caused by the threat of being in such a situation is indescribable and causes instant, terrible diarrhoea.'

Sex and relationships

In our study nearly half of our respondents (46 per cent) said IBS directly affected their sex lives. Sometimes IBS can make sex painful for both women and men:

'Painful sex with my husband was never really examined by doctors for IBS. I was told it was just one of those things,' says Tina, a 33-year-old who has had symptoms since she was twenty-five.

Other times the symptoms a person is suffering can take away all desire. Sex may also be affected by embarrassment, as Judy, a 41-year-old housewife who has had IBS for ten years, says:

'I worry that I might pass wind during intercourse. I was brought up to believe that passing wind just wasn't the thing to do and I get very embarrassed about it. Men make fun of it between themselves, but if a woman does it, it's a different thing.'

Andrea, a 26-year-old administrator who has suffered the condition since she was 13, says:

'Regrettably, I've never had the chance to find out if IBS would make sex painful for me. Apart from embarrassment, it often makes you feel too ill to care about the opposite sex.'

'I've never had a relationship as I never go out. By the evening I am in too much pain and bloated,' says Megan, a 42-year-old ex-teacher who has had IBS since she was twenty-one. Dorothy, an admin officer in her thirties who has had IBS ever since she can remember, finds sex painful:

'I have no partner at present. Most positions are painful. I only seem to be comfortable on my side with absolutely no pressure on my abdomen.'

And Rita, who has suffered from IBS for twenty-two years, says:

'Sex has for some time not been attempted for fear of being "caught out" at a highly personal moment in time but after twenty-four years of marriage, love, hugs and kisses make up for an awful lot of missed sex life!'

IBS often causes a lot of friction and tension between the sufferer and those with whom they live closely. This is almost inevitable unless the loved ones are particularly understanding – or suffer themselves! In extreme cases relationships are ruined and marriages break down. Gail remembers:

'I felt a failure in coping with IBS. When the children were small, and my husband's workload permitted a family outing, it always, so it seemed, "played up". He would say, "I knew this would happen," and I felt devastated. I did become depressed and anxious largely due to the IBS – not the other way round as my current GP imagined. I would go as far as to say I think it played a part in our consequent divorce.'

For Claudia, the worst occasion was:

'. . . when my husband's boss invited several people and their wives to his house for dinner and I just couldn't face the embarrassment of my stomach and refused to go. He went on his own and said I had to babysit for someone. I really felt I let him down and I'm sure his boss must have thought our marriage was on the rocks.'

IBS can also affect one's self-confidence, as Sarah, who is fifty-three and has had it since she was in her mid-thirties, writes:

'IBS has had a profound effect on my love life! I used to feel very sexually confident and outgoing. However, since developing IBS, I have had very few relationships and have become pretty reclusive. I have recently been contemplating the possibility of starting a new relationship with someone, but am very aware that embarrassment about wind etc. has left me feeling it's not worth going through all the anxiety, so I haven't done anything about pursuing the relationship.'

IBS has prevented Lorna from leaving her husband:

'My marriage is not terribly happy, and if I was "normal" I would probably have left my husband several years ago, but I don't have the courage to do so. He may have his faults, but he has always been absolutely super regarding my problems. He never minds how many times I need to visit the loo, and is very understanding. I feel it would be awful to have to start again with someone else, and try to explain. Imagine being with someone new, perhaps the first time you make love, then having to rush off to the loo! Also, if I left I would have nowhere to go. I would have to rent a flat or house, and I cannot afford it on what I earn. I could share with another girl if I were "normal" but I couldn't even think about sharing the way things are. So, I continue in a dead marriage. We don't argue a lot, I can't say it is stressful, we just live in the same house but don't communicate a lot. We have nothing in common, he goes out, I spend a lot of time on my own. I feel there is more to life than this, but what can I do about it?'

Lack of self-confidence can be a problem for men as well as women and Steven, a 24-year-old admin assistant, explains how he feels:

'I don't dare have a girlfriend. I lack self-confidence in that I'm dependent often on being near a toilet. I feel different, abnormal and frustrated in not being able to do what I want.'

Henry echoes Steven's sentiments.

'It makes it difficult to develop relationships with the opposite sex – what girl would want to go out with a man who daren't go out of reach of the loo? How can I be open with them about it?'

Maisie doesn't feel that her IBS has had any great effect on her relationships.

'I live alone and am not at present in a long-term relationship. I make a point of not telling new friends about my IBS. I want them to know me first as Maisie and not "the girl with the IBS". Nobody has run off yet when I've told them! I still have a lot of interest from men as I did before I got IBS and I'm glad to say I haven't lost interest in them!'

How work is affected

Maisie is thirty four and has had IBS for the past three years. Her working life as a civil servant has been severely affected, because pain prevents her from sitting down for more than ten minutes at a time.

'For the first seven months the pain was on and off. I underwent the usual medical tests which meant time off. My employers were very sympathetic. After seven months, the pain became and has remained continuous. Every minute of every day I'm either in bad or very bad pain and discomfort. There is no relief except for when I sleep.

'After seven months I decided to go on indefinite sick leave to concentrate all my energy into getting well. It was becoming impossible to do my job properly, as it entailed a lot of travelling and sitting in court and in interviews. Sitting had become, and still is, unbearably uncomfortable. I have reached the stage now where most of my day is spent either on the move or standing up. That's not to say that I'm in very much less discomfort when I'm on the move, it's just more easy to bear, pacing about.

After the hospitals had told her they couldn't help any more, Maisie decided to try alternative medicine. She spent £1000 on trying to find a cure but nothing helped even in the slightest. Her symptoms gradually got worse. She continues:

'After seven months of being on sick leave, I had a chat with my boss and decided to accept a completely different job. I had got worse while I was on sick leave but as I couldn't see an end to this problem I knew I just had to go back to survive. I don't just mean financially – but I couldn't afford to give in to it.

'The job I do now is very much less demanding. It enables me to walk around a fair bit but at the end of the day it is still a desk job and I'm just so uncomfortable sitting down that I can't concentrate.

'I'm unhappy and frustrated at work now. Every day I don't feel well enough to go in but I make myself. I haven't missed a day since I went back two years ago but there are times when I've had to continue work lying on the floor in pain. When I get home I give myself a pat on the back for getting through the day. Very occasionally I allow myself a good cry, take a deep breath and start again. There is never a morning when I don't wake up full of renewed hope that maybe today's the day.

'I'm three years behind as far as promotion is concerned and it is very frustrating seeing my contemporaries pass me by. Having said that, IBS has made me take stock of my life and sort out my priorities. I value my health, family and friends even more now.'

Maisie is tired of the daily struggle and is considering a complete change of career. She explains it this way:

'If a typist loses her arm she doesn't go back to typing – she sits down and thinks what else she can do with what she has left. Maybe it is time for me to accept that I have got a disability which prevents me from doing a desk job. Also, so much of my energy goes into battling against IBS that I don't currently need such a demanding job. Doing routine work stretches me. I'm trying to do something which I'm not fit to do and this is causing me stress and in turn must be affecting my IBS.'

Maisie's decision not to apply for promotion because she needs all her energy to cope with IBS has meant loss of pride and self-esteem.

Sheila is a finance clerk and she's had IBS for five years. Her main symptom is severe bloating and wind. She describes what it's like at work:

'I'd love to change my job but don't know how I would cope as I spend so much time in the toilet. It's difficult now at work with people noticing. I spend most of my time lying on the floor trying to pass wind or bent double in pain. I have to hold or suppress the symptoms, which makes it worse, or keep going out to the toilet. I am worried about how I can hold a job down in this condition. It's becoming increasingly difficult for me to hide the symptoms.'

At the moment Sheila is off work.

Rita is forty-four and works as a local government officer. This year she has lost three months due to her IBS. She suffers from continuous diarrhoea and abdominal pain.

'Travelling to work is a major problem on bad days – I am in constant fear of any hold-up in transport in case I need to rush to the toilet. Sitting in on meetings or even travelling to them is also a problem. What if I need to leave in a hurry and cannot find the cloakroom? (I usually arrive extra early and try to do this first!)

'Part of my job is to meet and talk to the public, which I usually find rewarding, but not feeling 100 per cent for the best part of my working day causes stress; I feel as if I am on stage, and put on my best face and performance for my customers, the public. Career promotion has twice been put on one side as I was unable to fulfil the obligations of the posts offered, because of IBS. If you are working as a team, you cannot expect your colleagues to cover or carry you for long periods. This again I feel stressed and angry about – angry with myself for not being in control. My present head of section has always been very kind and thoughtful about my condition but when he leaves later on this year I fear his replacement will not be so easy. I have already had the unkind remarks about people pulling their weight etc!'

For those sufferers whose symptoms are worse in the morning, nine-to-five jobs can be very difficult. Edwina has always suffered with her bowels but did not worry too much about it until she started working in an office.

'I was working in a bingo hall where I didn't have to be in work until 1 pm and that gave me the time to go to the loo as many times as I needed. It was when I got into the claustrophobic office atmosphere that the symptoms really flared up. I was getting up at 6.30 am and still going to the loo at 9 am. It would start with windy crampy pains and spasms that would double me over. Then the stools would start. When I thought the bowel was empty the whole process would begin again, sometimes up to eight or nine times in the morning, maybe more. Luckily, my work was on flexi-time but I was finding it hard to make it for 9.30 am. I would put my coat on to leave and have to rush back to the loo. It was the same at work. By 10 am, my stomach would be empty and the foul wind would start. I would then have to think of excuses to leave the office and rush to the loo. I had to start going home at lunchtime as I could not eat at work because as soon as I did the wind would begin again. My work did suffer. I was warned about my sick leave and was in constant debit with my flexi-time.

'The symptoms were often accompanied by hot flushes and panic attacks, especially in pubs, shops, buses and in the office. When I'm out I need my space – claustrophobia brings my symptoms on.

'At Christmas I went to my doctor and asked for a sick note, as I felt so bad I think if I had continued working I would have had a nervous breakdown. I was physically and mentally exhausted with the whole thing. My employers, the Department of Social Security, were very good. They sent a welfare officer every month to see how I was and to offer advice. By the September I decided to resign as I could not see myself returning and I have been on Invalidity Benefit ever since. I'm feeling better now I'm at home but if I have to go anywhere like the doctor's or for a night out, the severe symptoms begin again.

For Adele, who has had IBS for nine years, the pressure of work aggravated her symptoms.

'I became a temporary veterinary nurse, a job I had not done for twelve years and a solo position as opposed to a team one as I had done previously. I found the vet I worked for very abrupt and unfriendly, with very high standards. Before operations were due to begin each morning I frequently had to go to the loo with diarrhoea.'

At present she is a part-time youth and community worker and goes on to say:

'I have had diarrhoea before leaving home for difficult meetings which seems daft, but I am OK once I get there. It is a job which I enjoy and I am determined not to let my IBS stop me.'

Even working from home isn't without its problems, as Brenda, a 63-year-old writer, explains:

'I can't leave the house before 10 am. This interferes with professional appointments, conferences etc. I have two to four wasted hours daily because of urgent visits to the lavatory, 6 to 10 am.'

Giving up work

Nearly 5 per cent of those taking part in our survey were unable to work at all because of their symptoms.

Amy has tried everything over the last twenty years in the hope of finding a cure. She had to give up her job as a teacher and is no longer able to work, but her enforced rest hasn't eased the symptoms. When she was working she was off continually and is now on Invalidity Benefit. She says:

'I am very slow and get tired easily. I am always battling against the pain. There is so much I want to do but the pain stops me.'

Being unable to work has meant lack of money and an insecurity that causes anxiety, and also prevents her from doing things she would like to.

Andrea also had to give up her job and now works from home in a family business:

'Despite a fairly positive attitude to "making the best of it", I have found my working life very curtailed, right from having to drop out of doing science A Levels because I was too ill to concentrate properly. I was an able student but have had to adapt to doing what my body is capable of rather than my mind.'

Graham is fifty-six and was a milkman for twenty-four years. He enjoyed the work, being outside in the fresh air, meeting people every day and, best of all, being able to plan the workload to suit himself. After an operation for haemorrhoids, he found that he had trouble with diarrhoea. He went to the doctor and, after having to undergo various investigations, was told that he 'probably had' IBS, as they couldn't find anything wrong! He was prescribed anti-diarrhoeal drug.

'I was able to carry on with my outside job, although I had to be aware of the locations of all the toilets on my round. I found that I needed to go while working more and more often,' he says.

He coped for quite a long time, but in October 1990 had very severe stomach pains that kept him off work for five weeks. It was found that he had a disease of the small intestine which cleared up with antibiotics. The following February he was off work for a further three weeks. Various tests were given, including ones for food allergies, but all were negative. By October his condition had worsened and he was forced to stop work.

'During one of my frequent visits, my GP told me, "You will have to accept that you may be unable to continue with your outside job, and should ask your employers if they are able to offer you an inside job." This wasn't possible and it was suggested that I apply for early retirement.'

At the time of writing Graham is on sick pay, but his employer is trying to hasten his retirement.

Mick is fifty five and has suffered from constipation for many years. For sixteen years he took a laxative that his doctor assured him had no long-term ill-effects. When he started to get pains in his right abdomen his doctor decided perhaps he should not be taking the laxative after all. Eventually IBS was diagnosed. Mick remembers how, six years ago, the doctor advised him to give up work.

'My doctor suggested it would be advisable for me to give up work in view of my continued ill health, and as my job was stressful this would help my condition. After six years of being home with no stress (except the illness), I have continued to gradually get worse and life has become a misery only consoled by a loving and considerate family without whose help I could not cope. I gave up a successful career with excellent prospects.'

What follows is an upsetting account of how ignorance and intolerance have forced Lorna to leave two jobs.

'I was getting very depressed and bored at home after my family left home and my marriage was going through a sticky patch. I had had IBS problems for many years though didn't at the time know what the problem was, medically speaking. I decided to get a job.

'I went back to teaching for one year but found it too stressful. I then got a post at a local government office. It soon became obvious that some of my work colleagues found me smelly. I have very bad wind problems which I cannot always control. Some people with very sensitive noses seemed to find me offensive all the time – my bowel doesn't empty properly and this may be the problem here. They would make remarks which I tried to ignore. The office employed more than 500 people and as the months passed I became an office joke with one or two little references in notes and even snide remarks in the office newsletter.

'I sought medical help but this only seemed to make matters worse. I didn't want to be beaten by the problem but in the end I had to give up the job after eighteen months for my own sanity.

'I then found a job doing individual coaching with children at a private school. I enjoyed the work but there were only two staff loos in the school and this caused me problems as they were often both engaged. There was also one member of staff with a particularly sensitive nose – there always is! – and she made sure everyone knew of my problem. The stress, of course, made the problem even worse and I started to avoid contact with the other staff as much as possible. After three and a half years I finally gave up and left. I now am back at home!'

Many readers will feel sympathy with Lorna and anger at the way she was treated. The general public need educating about IBS so that this kind of thing doesn't happen.

Having IBS can prevent people from taking up jobs they would like. Louise wanted to take up nursing but realized her guts would never cope with the shift system and the stress of the job. IBS kept Rosemary at home once her children grew up when she would have liked to return to work. Claudia had hoped to study at university and go on to get a good job but IBS put paid to her plans and she had to leave school early.

'I worked in a shop for about a year. I eventually plucked up the courage to get a better job, but I had to be very choosy. It had to be one where there was always noise to hide my tummy noises, and where I was free to go to the loo without being too obvious. I worked in a building society. This was fine until I progressed to being a cashier when I was caught in the trap again; as soon as I had a customer and thousands of pounds waiting to be counted I was churning inside again and physically almost sick trying to get through to the end of the transaction. I eventually left the building society with "nerves" again.

'I had a year off work hoping relaxation might help. I was very frustrated. I knew I was capable of using my mind but my body wouldn't let me.

'After my year off I got a job in an office (carefully planned for noise and escape routes). This was fine but as I was promoted I had to attend meetings and that was impossible, so I managed to coincide that with being able to start a family and escaped that one.

Time off from work, not only due to the symptoms but also visits to the doctor, hospital and other health professionals, can mount up.

'Fortunately, I am self-employed; the scores of working hours I have lost, in the recent past, is distressing and frustrating to me, but would presumably have been more so to an employer!' *says Sean.*

It is very important that employers recognize IBS as a debilitating illness. As there is still much ignorance surrounding the condition, you are lucky if those you work with are understanding. Bernard has twice suffered at the hands of unsympathetic employers.

'The stomach problems in 1987 were probably the result of stress caused by marital problems which have considerably worsened since then. It was from 1987 that my health worsened to such a degree that it necessitated me having sick leave and my situation was not helped by a very unsympathetic employer who was apparently suggesting that I was malingering by my absence.'

Eventually, after having worked for this firm for a number of years, he was made redundant, although he considers that he was sacked. Next, after passing the examination and declaring he had IBS, he found work with the Inland Revenue. By this time his health had considerably worsened.

'I had had little in the way of sick leave but certain members of management were keeping check of my visits to the toilet. I was finding it difficult to give of my best with all of these pressures.'

Finally, the Inland Revenue terminated his employment. Since then, Bernard has been registered as disabled with anxiety and depression.

Domestic Life

Tiredness, lethargy and pain can affect housework as they do other activities. Tasks are made slower and more difficult or they may not be possible at all. Joyce worries that she neglects her children because she spends so much time on the toilet.

Shopping can be difficult for those of us who need to be near a toilet. Some people only shop during pub opening hours so that their facilities can be used; others stick to one shop. Some people cannot go shopping at all. Queueing can often be a problem; several sufferers mention having to leave the queue to go to the toilet quickly.

Travel

A vast number of IBS sufferers say that travelling is restricted – nearly 70 per cent in our study. Both long-distance and short everyday journeys can cause all sorts of problems for the IBS sufferer. As Malcolm says: 'I need to find out where the toilets are before I travel anywhere.'

Motorway travel and traffic jams can be a source of anxiety and some people can never travel by public transport – although those who need toilets nearby often feel better on trains or planes.

The daily journey to work can be quite harrowing for some people. Rita goes by car:

'Travel puts the fear into me, even the 15-minute journey to work

– what could happen if the car breaks down or an accident causes delay etc? I try not to think too much about it but I have been caught out once too often.'

Julie's IBS restricts her travel greatly. She lives in London and usually travels by bus.

'After a couple of narrow escapes on the Underground, when I had to ask to use the staff loos, I am now scared stiff to go on the tube. The thought of getting stuck between stations acts as an instant enema, yet before I got IBS I travelled everywhere by Underground without giving it a second thought.'

Travelling abroad may be impossible or only undertaken with difficulty. Brenda says that for her:

'Travel abroad is out, my gut keeps Greenwich Meantime! I can only visit where there is more than one loo. No journey can start before 10 am.'

Sheila says:

'I've been abroad this year and it was horrendous, being cramped in an aircraft with a stomach like a balloon and pressure in the cabin making the symptoms worse. I could have gone mad.'

Social life

Dealing with the effects of long-term IBS becomes a way of life. It is not unusual for all a sufferer's activities to be arranged around her or his symptoms. It can seriously restrict people's lives.

Rita describes how it has affected her:

'For nearly eight months last year I only went to work, to the village or stayed at home, and it was not much of a life. In desperation I even asked for my gut to be removed and a bag attached to let me live a better form of life, but that was greeted with horror by my doctor.

'I no longer go on holiday, out for the day, on theatre trips etc. My husband has been long-suffering – we do disagree about the way it affects our lives but he has also been very understanding. Our social life has been greatly reduced, as sickness, diarrhoea and pain has a disastrous effect on it.'

As Rita says, IBS restricts where she is able to go. It can sometimes cause a sufferer to be unable to leave the house at all. Amy is almost a recluse because of the wind she suffers. Andrea has been agoraphobic for five years, since she was twenty-one:

'It began when I started to suffer constantly from severe pain and nausea. I am working on it but I don't go far from home at present. Shopping is very difficult. My life is severely restricted. IBS has caused the agoraphobia and compounded the problem. But I'm resourceful and I'm not going to give up trying to improve the situation.'

Claudia finds that every part of her life is affected.

'Everyday life is ruined. I can't even sleep without being troubled. We have to have the TV on at meal times to disguise my stomach noises or I am dashing to the loo. I make excuses not to go to friends' houses for coffee, not to join any groups or societies, not to go to any meetings. Even going to the library is an ordeal. I dread being a passenger in a car and having to wait for someone to stop talking or get out before the engine starts again. I dread being caught in a conversation in a corridor or a shop. I always have to keep myself busy dashing around so that I have an excuse not to be caught. And underneath, I am so tired and would love to do all the things I am running away from.'

Invariably people with IBS say they cope by taking each day at a time. Forward planning is often impossible, as Megan explains:

I don't like letting people down, but being constantly unwell you have to keep cancelling arrangements.'

The tiredness that sometimes accompanies IBS can prevent people from doing what they want, and other symptoms can also be restrictive. Fiona, a 23-year-old student, says:

'Sometimes if my stomach is bloated I don't feel able to do my exercise class or go swimming – it makes me too self-conscious.'

And Judy says:

'Most leisure activities take part in the evening and I don't usually feel very good then so I don't go out.'

'IBS has really dominated my life to such an extent that I have given up on going to the theatre, given up on evening classes and as for exams, well, forget it! I spent more time in the loo than in the exam hall, an experience I would not like to repeat!'

says Audrey, who suffers particularly from severe bloating after a meal and often an urgent need to go to the toilet. Because she has to dash to the toilet before breakfast it makes staying in a hotel or with friends unbearable for her.

Ruby, who has had IBS for five years, says:

'I cannot go on holiday easily now as I'm always afraid of soiling clothes or bedclothes.'

Sheila feels that because of her symptoms she is 'totally unacceptable socially'.

Ida is seventy-six, and has been discouraged by other people's attitudes:

'I have been very active and gone dancing for years, but the past years I have felt a nuisance. People don't understand. I felt they thought I was making a mountain out of molehill, so I have given up dancing.'

Ingrid is seventy-seven. Some days she spends two hours making frequent visits to the lavatory. She finds it usually occurs when she is active in the garden or doing the heavier housework and it has meant that she cannot enjoy her hobby of walking.

'The distressing time occurs when I'm out walking or shopping. I have only a few minutes' warning and must find a toilet. On several occasions I have not arrived in time, much to my distress. I have coped with this by cutting out walking in the country and trying at all times to be within easy reach of a toilet.'

IBS can even affect the clothes a person wears. Maisie, who suffers from severe abdominal pain, says:

'I can't wear any fitted clothing, not even loose elastic, because it makes my symptoms worse. I can't therefore wear skirts or trousers, nor even tights or some swimsuits. This breaks my heart because I love clothes and it makes me feel good to look good. However, with some careful shopping, I've come up with some good alternatives – dress suits, hold-up stockings, cat suits etc.'

And Sarah explains how it has affected what she has been able to wear over the seventeen years she has had IBS.

'When I first began to suffer from it really severely I would go to work in the jeans I had been accustomed to wearing for years, but would find that by about lunchtime I was having to go home and change into skirts with baggy tops to try to hide my huge distended stomach. Eventually I had to more or less change my style of clothing and the size of my wardrobe to cope with the fact that I could no longer tolerate anything around my stomach and waist that was even slightly fitting. It profoundly shook my self-esteem and sense of self-identity as my body image completely changed. I also stopped being able to exercise as much as I had been accustomed to and this added to my increasing size. Fortunately, after about a couple of years, baggy trousers became fashionable and I was able to go back to wearing pants again which restored some of my old sense of identity.

'It has taken years for me to begin to feel really comfortable with my body again. And it's only in the last three to four years, since I have learned to control my IBS, by taking care about my diet, that I have felt comfortable to start exercising again. It was just too painful before.'

Some people may also be restricted in eating out, socializing and travelling because of the diet they are following. Some of the diets thought to help IBS such as gluten-free and anti-candida diets and those that avoid potential allergens, can drastically reduce the foods and drinks a person is able to consume. You may also suffer from loss of appetite or only be able to tolerate small meals. You may be in pain after eating. You may need to go to the toilet after eating, or during a meal, which can be restrictive and embarrassing. In fact, your enjoyment of food can be thoroughly ruined. Julie describes her diet as 'gluten-free, caffeine-free, dairy-free, red meat-free, fun-free!'

Not everyone, however, leads a limited life. Maria, who is fifty-eight and has had IBS for two years, says:

'I don't let it affect my work or my leisure. I get on with my life and carry on regardless.'

A study done in London discovered that over 40 per cent of the patients who took part were affected by their IBS in the areas of work, travel, socializing, sexual intercourse, domestic and leisure activities, food and eating with others.[2] Women were more likely to be disabled by their symptoms and their sex lives were more likely to be affected. The study found that women, on the whole, were more seriously affected by their IBS than men. The question remains as to whether women are more easily incapacitated by their symptoms or whether their symptoms are actually worse than men's – or even, are women more ready to admit to symptoms, especially psychological ones?

The above study is the only one we have come across in our research for this book that looks at how the lives of people with IBS are affected, and even this one does not go into much detail. While there are many studies that examine the possible causes of IBS and the psychological make-up of the sufferer, this book is the first time that the physical and psychological consequences of living with the condition have been looked at in any depth.

IBS can have various other physical effects in addition to the well-known symptoms. Janet, a 48-year-old credit control clerk who has suffered from the condition for twenty-two years, has a deep pain in the left groin that affects the muscle and has made walking difficult, at times impossible. Osteopathy has made the muscle more supple and has helped her to walk more easily, but she still has attacks when she needs to use a stick.

Living with IBS

It must be said that although the consequences of living with IBS that are described in this chapter make depressing reading, most people do not experience such a severe effect on their lives. This chapter is, in part, a reflection of our sample of sufferers. Those people with IBS whose lives are not seriously affected were much less likely to write to us about their experiences.

When one of the authors (Susan Backhouse) was first diagnosed as having a spastic colon twenty-two years ago, few people had heard of it. She suspected then that the term didn't mean much, but was simply describing a symptom. Even today, IBS needs to be more fully recognized by those in the medical profession and the general public. More acknowledgement needs to be given to the pain and distress those with IBS may suffer, and more information needs to be available about self-help methods while the medical profession can offer us so little. People with IBS need to get together and talk to each other. Finding ways that have helped someone else may help you. Talking to others with the condition, especially if you've been newly diagnosed or have spent years not knowing of anyone else with IBS, can be a liberating experience! Reassurance and affirmation can work a lot better than anti-spasmodics and bulking agents, although maybe you will want the lot! Most importantly, sufferers should not be made to feel it's their fault, or that 'it's all in the mind'.

Andrea says:

'Having IBS makes me angry and resentful. I am frustrated by the restriction and angry about people's attitude to it. Anger is very bad for your health and it doesn't help your guts! Society should not blame people for becoming ill, it is not something that happens by "incorrect thinking" or subconscious choice.'

The final word goes to Maisie.

'IBS is one long nightmare. To me, it is like being stuck in a tunnel. All the lights have gone out and the communication system is not working. You do not know why the train has stopped and what is wrong with it and nobody can tell you because the intercom system has failed. You are sitting in darkness and can see no light at the end of the tunnel. However, deep down, however frightened you are, you know that you will eventually get out. It's just a matter of when.'

Chapter 5

Coming to Terms with It

'Nothing has helped my IBS except my own attempts to remain calm and not let tension build up. I try to make contact with as many people as I can and help them in whatever way I can. When I start to feel I am being creative and fulfilling my potential in some way, I feel altogether different.'

IBS often makes sufferers feel out of control of their bodies and out of control of their lives. Probably the most crucial aspect of coping with it is regaining that feeling of control. This chapter looks at the many different ways that people with IBS are attempting to do just that.

Coping with IBS as a child

Some people don't realize they have IBS until they have suffered its symptoms for a long time, either because the medical professionals haven't diagnosed it as such or because they haven't sought medical help at all. For some sufferers, symptoms begin during childhood.

One of the authors (Susan Backhouse) recalls:

'For many years I was unaware that other people suffered in the way that I did. I first remember the symptoms occurring when I was twelve, but I didn't go to the doctor until I was fifteen. By then, I was affected every day and my life was very much tied up with coping with the symptoms. As a girl and young woman who didn't talk to anyone at all about it, the coping option open to me was mainly trying to avoid situations where I couldn't go to the toilet whenever I needed to – not easy, as children's lives are usually controlled by various adults. I would "skive off"; pretend to be ill; dose myself up with kaolin and morphine (I never got constipated!);

try not to let people know I was going to the toilet in case I needed to go again soon and they commented on it. I consciously avoided people and situations that made me feel restricted and out of control. I developed, in all other aspects of my life, an attitude that nothing was worth worrying about; if it happened then I'd cope. All my energies were, instead, devoted to the anxiety about not being able to get to the toilet in time!'

Coping with IBS is hard for anyone who doesn't know that others have it but it is especially hard for children and young adults because they have less control over their lives.

Coping with the medical profession

Sarah, who has suffered for seventeen years, feels optimistic that her IBS will improve. She can go for long pain-free periods now, though she used to be permanently in pain. She believes it is necessary to stop looking to the medical profession and says it would help if there were a more open attitude from doctors, who should be prepared to accept their ignorance of many things instead of implying that their patients are hypochondriacs.

Many of us have been brought up to have a lot of faith in the mainstream medical profession. Doctors are often looked up to and few of us question their competence. After all, they are the experts. They have the knowledge and the power. One of the problems with this is that we don't learn to take responsibility for our own health; we are too dependent on doctors and the prescriptions they give us. Another problem is that as patients we can be made to feel IBS is 'our fault' and that we're wasting the doctors' time asking for help with this condition. Some doctors may hide their ignorance by making their patients feel their complaint is unimportant. You may find that you know more about IBS than your GP!

Sarah says:

'The bowel specialist said I should be ashamed of wasting everybody's valuable time and . . . I was obsessed with my bowels. I never was told I had IBS in those early years. I went to a medical library and started taking responsibility for my own health.'

She felt what she needed most when she first sought help was

87

someone consistent who would have 'stayed with her' until the problem was discovered and treated instead of being sent from one person to another and having to start all over again each time.

Sometimes doctors can trivialize the patient's problem. Connie is in her twenties and has been unable to work for fifteen months because of her IBS. She says:

'I truly believe that my condition has been made worse by local doctors and specialists I have seen, as their general attitude has been "go away and forget about it and it will go away". One doctor told me to have a baby and that would clear me out – I wonder if anyone else has tried this!?'

It is because, at present, the mainstream medical profession seems to offer so little to people with IBS that sufferers have to find their own ways of coping with it. Many sufferers want to be able to take responsibility for themselves because, as one put it, 'it makes me feel less of a victim'. The need for self-help groups is especially apparent. (See p. 100.) Reading as much as possible about the condition is one way of finding out more information and attempting to take control again. However, until recently there has been very little available to the lay person on the subject. (See Appendix I for a book list.)

A large number of people try alternative (or complementary) medicine, in spite of this often being very expensive. The range of disciplines that are tried includes homeopathy, acupuncture, herbalism, osteopathy, naturopathy, reflexology, autogenics, massage, colonic irrigation, Alexander technique, hypnotherapy, aromatherapy, and iridology. There doesn't appear to be any one particular technique that is especially beneficial to IBS and people often try several before they find one that helps, if indeed any do. However, some types of alternative medicine do seem to significantly reduce certain symptoms and, of course, there is less worry about side-effects and dependency. (See Chapter 3.)

Sarah, whose main symptoms are pain and bloating, together with constipation alternating with diarrhoea, explains how she copes:

'For a long time I tried to get help from the medical profession but was so appalled with the attitudes I came across that I started to seek help from the 'alternative' health care movement. I tried acupuncture, massage and so forth, which were some help, but eventually I found that a combination of therapy and reading widely to develop my own dietary regime were the things that have most reduced the stress of it. However, if I have an attack before or around social events I still find it very stressful, although I can usually reduce the attack considerably by drinking lots of camomile tea and live goat's milk yoghurt. Knowing that this really does work for me has been a big help in reducing the related stress and anxiety.'

Coping with pain

Abdominal pain is the most commonly reported symptom and it is believed to be the one that is most likely to cause people to seek help from the medical profession. A study conducted in London among hospital outpatients with IBS found that half of those taking part were in pain for more than three hours a day, over half for twenty one or more days in a month and just under half experienced 'marked or severe' pain.[1] It is no wonder people seek help!

Sean is in his forties with two teenage sons. He has been suffering from painful IBS attacks for five years.

'When in severe pain – I judge that it's severe, because I know from experience that my pain-toleration threshold is quite high – I supplement the anti-spasmodic drugs with soluble aspirin, which seems, anyway, more quick-acting and effective than anything!'

He goes on to describe the pain he experiences.

'It varies in intensity from a mere niggling and persistent discomfort sometimes felt in the stomach, sometimes in the back and sometimes even in the shoulder blades to a grand series of contraction-like pains which reduce me to lying flat on the floor – and this position sometimes helps the attack to pass. During the attacks I feel slightly faint and nauseous, and I find it virtually impossible to concentrate on anything until the worst is over, which transpires after taking an anti-spasmodic or aspirin (or both) but sometimes spontaneously, the pain going as quickly as it came.'

Ingrid suffers from severe abdominal swelling 'to the size of a football', wind and pain.

'I've had so many tablets and none of them have been any help at all. The only way to relieve the pain and swelling for me is to lie down with a hot-water bottle on the area and stay there overnight. By morning I am usually back to my normal size again and the pain has gone.'

Felicity has found that the pain she suffers has become particularly vicious since she had an operation to have her spleen removed. She has found that massage helps.

'When in the middle of the pain I get my husband to massage my back from the hips upwards. It seems to alleviate the pain. He does that about twice a day. I haven't yet found any of the tablets I've been prescribed any use.'

If you have ever been told that your complaints about your pains were due to your having a 'low tolerance' of pain (meaning that your pains are probably not that bad, it's just that you complain of them more!) it may be encouraging to know that a study done in 1987 found that IBS sufferers were able to tolerate pain a lot better than people without IBS.[2] IBS and non-IBS people had to undergo various painful tests. The former reported less pain than the latter, and reported the pain a lot later.

Pain should not be ignored – it is the way our bodies tell us that something is wrong. If you have an injured knee, for instance, you may relieve the pain by taking painkillers but there may then be a temptation to treat it as you would a normal knee while it still needs a chance to heal. Similarly, with abdominal pain, it is important to remember that pain is a symptom of your malfunctioning digestive system. If possible, give your body a chance to deal with pain itself. The more you use drugs as painkillers the more the production of the body's natural painkillers, endorphins, will be reduced and they will become less effective. You are more likely to feel pain if you are tense, so learning to relax your mind and body will help. A hot-water bottle wrapped in a towel and held on the abdomen is a good way to ease pain; rubbing, stroking and gently pressing the painful area may also help by inhibiting the passage of nerve impulses and triggering the production of pain-relieving hormones.

Marie Langley runs an organisation called Unwind – a non-profit-making self-help group for people who suffer from pain in all its forms: physical, mental and emotional (see p. 149 for address). Through her own experiences of pain and her studies into pain control techniques, she has developed several self-help programmes on tape to help people deal with their pain.

She tells us that helplessness makes pain more overwhelming. Her programmes are aimed at achieving a feeling of control over the pain. Because the way we think has such an influence over the perception of pain, positive thinking is very important.

Keeping morale up

Sometimes coping is an attitude of mind. Many people with IBS report that they keep busy to put it out of their minds and they feel dwelling on it too much makes it worse. For Maisie, it is important that she tries to remain optimistic that things will change for the better.

'My symptoms have got steadily worse. I'm an optimistic person by nature; I only hope I don't run out of optimism before I'm better. I think mental attitude is very important, but if that's the case, I can't understand how I have not been successful in willing myself better! I cope by being positive, optimistic and never giving up the battle. Occasionally, I allow myself a good cry but then I feel better for it and ready to fight another day.

'I socialize with friends regularly. The way I look at it is I'd rather be in pain in a restaurant with friends than in pain looking at the four walls at home. A sense of humour is a great asset to have if you're suffering from IBS. Unfortunately, cinema, theatre, concerts etc. are a thing of the past. So is travel. I just can't bear the discomfort of sitting through it. Having said that, I do put up with it in restaurants and in friends' houses but the mental effort I have to put in knocks me out.'

Julie copes by

'not forcing myself to do things I really don't want to do and not feeling guilty about it.

'I suffered terrible IBS only twelve months ago, but now I have learned to control the symptoms considerably by calming down and cutting out the anxiety which is my main problem. Now I can feel an attack coming on and can control it so that my symptoms do not get too distressing.'

Lily, a 47-year-old farmer's wife, says:

'I try not to get angry and upset about things that don't matter that much. I try not to lose my temper. I try to take each day as it comes. If I were calmer I think my IBS would go.'

Chrystal believes that she would have coped better in a past generation when life wasn't so hectic. Maureen, a 40-year-old shop assistant and housewife says:

'I've taken time to be me and to be quiet.'

And Sarah says

'I think having a strong, positive personality has helped me to survive IBS.'

Louise states:

'I have to get up early to deal with my two to three trips to the loo, then I try to forget about it for the rest of the day.'

Brenda makes it clear to colleagues that she may have to break appointments or be late for them. Almost invariably, people with IBS say the way they cope is to take one day at a time. George says:

'I know if I only go to the loo once in the morning it's going to be a "good" day.'

Tricia tells her story and how she copes:

'I have suffered from IBS for the past seven years and know what utter misery it can bring.

'Mine started innocently enough after a meal out with friends. Half an hour after leaving the restaurant I developed violent diarrhoea and had to ask them to stop the car several times on the journey home so that I could dash into a field. This was dreadfully embarrassing, but luckily I knew them well.

'At first, I never really gave it another thought, presuming it was a touch of food poisoning, but later I began to be concerned about it happening again. This fear grew and grew over the following months until after about a year I was terrified to leave the house. I couldn't even walk to the post office, five minutes away. The only journey I could manage was to work and back – four miles.

Anything more than that and I would break out into a cold sweat, have palpitations, violent stomach cramps and instant diarrhoea. Shopping at the weekend had to be accomplished within pub hours so that I could use their facilities.

'Eventually I knew I had to seek professional help before I became completely housebound. A pharmacist friend suggested I try an anti-diarrhoeal drug and to my intense relief I found it worked perfectly. At first I would take six a day, then stop for a couple of days as I found I would become constipated. I talked over the problem with my doctor, who was quite understanding and gave me the drug on prescription. He also suggested a psychologist might help. I was a bit wary of this but it turned out to be the first step on the road to recovery.

'The lady he sent me to was wonderful. She explained what was happening to my body and why and made me keep a graph of my stress levels. She also taught me the art of relaxation. After a dozen or so appointments I felt I was able to cope on my own. The only time I reach for the anti-diarrhoeal drug now is if I am going on a journey of any length. I even manage to go on foreign holidays without too much anguish. I never leave the house without a few capsules in my handbag, but I find that a pack of twelve will last me three months or more.

'Relaxation tapes played through headphones at night just before you go to sleep are wonderfully soothing. I also leave affirmations around the house and in the car, such as "Do the thing you fear and death of fear is certain" and "My stomach muscles are smooth and soft". Anything really that reminds me to relax my tummy muscles.

'I am fine until someone suggests a sudden journey and I haven't had time to prepare with my anti-diarrhoeal drug – I take two capsules two hours before I need to leave and that keeps me loo-free for twenty four hours. It's almost as if someone kicks me in the stomach and I can feel the message whiz down my bowel, my heart thumps and I begin to panic. If I can get out of the situation I will and have made some bizarre excuses, knowing that people are thinking I've gone completely off my head.

'I am quite sure that no one thing cures IBS. It has to be a combination of sensible eating, self-awareness, exercise and relaxation, and understanding relatives and friends.'

Nicola recounts her story:

'I was first diagnosed as being an IBS sufferer seven years ago by what I now realize was a surprisingly sympathetic and knowledgeable doctor who took a very matter-of-fact approach to my symptoms. Having just experienced the most excruciating stomach cramps that left me doubled up in pain and breathless, I was amazed to be told, "Spastic colon, not surprising given what you've been through, let's try you on an anti-spasmodic." So from being totally ignorant of the existence of IBS I was suddenly pitched into a new period of my life as an "IBS sufferer". I remember feeling an overwhelming sense of relief – at least now I had a name for the pain, and I wasn't dying of cancer – in fact I wasn't dying at all! I consider myself to be very lucky. My doctor's manner was so pragmatic, briefly explaining the possible causes and treatments, recommending certain diets, that I instinctively adopted the same approach. This, coupled with the fact that few of my friends and relatives had ever heard of the disease, led me to treat it with a degree of indifference that I still advocate today.

'On a practical level I know that I may well experience the symptoms, so I carry my survival kit with me (anti-spasmodics and a high-fibre biscuit) but by doing that I feel that I have some control over my life, which seems to reduce the likelihood of an attack. Furthermore, I've learnt to identify what might be called "risky" times – stressful situations that are at first glance uncontrollable (the obnoxious colleague at work who makes your life miserable, the boyfriend who's too demanding, the next job interview) but which when I think about them can be broken down into more manageable and therefore controllable chunks. In addition, for the last five years I've been meditating, a practice I thoroughly recommend – somehow it puts everything into perspective, reduces my feelings of anxiety and, increasingly, the frequency of my attacks/symptoms.

'Over the last few years I have become increasingly aware of, and surprised by, the number of friends who have developed IBS. Often their stories have elements in common with mine – a traumatic life event (in my case the loss of my partner) followed a few weeks later by spiralling anxiety and the dreaded stomach cramps. Unlike me, however, most fellow-sufferers that I know still have violent and debilitating symptoms that don't seem to respond to any of the treatments. I see myself as one of the IBS survivors. Perhaps my experiences will give others some hope? My life isn't all pain, doom and gloom, ruled by this mythical beast. In fact I thoroughly enjoy my life and feel I have control over my IBS and not the other way round. It's not all pain, and it's not fatal, there are practical ways of dealing with it.'

Lucy, who has had IBS for fourteen years, has recently returned from a year travelling abroad during which she surprised herself with what she was able to do.

'It took me a long time to agree to give up my security of a flat, a job, family and friends and to go travelling in Central America and Mexico for a year.

'There were so many other things to worry about that I didn't spend too much time worrying about the problems of having IBS while on the other side of the world. One fact comforted me – the guide books told me that everyone who visits Mexico is troubled by the dreaded "Montezuma's Revenge", so I wouldn't be the only one dashing to the toilet.

'To be honest, if I'd known exactly what was in store for me I either wouldn't have gone or else I'd have worried so much I'd have made myself quite ill. What I hadn't anticipated was the bus journeys (the only way for people on our budget to get around). Generally these were between seven and fourteen hours and sometimes up to twenty four hours. Toilets on board were almost unheard of and almost always locked when they did feature. I never once checked if one was open in case I found it locked and ended up panicking. The buses would generally stop every four or five hours (less often if it was a night bus) for half an hour. The worry here would be being able to go to the toilet once if necessary and not set my bowels off so they would want to go ten more times. The other worry was that the bus would take off, leaving me stranded without my luggage, or my boyfriend, in the middle of nowhere. I won't say much about the toilets other than if you've gotta go you've gotta go – no seats, often no doors, no water, no paper, lots of cockroaches, spiders and lizards.

'The routine prior to a bus journey was to eat very little for twenty four hours beforehand, to go to the toilet as much as possible before leaving the hotel, then to take one or two codeine phosphate tablets or anti-diarrhoeal capsules one hour before the journey. The difficulty is taking the right dose so that the bowel is stopped for twenty four hours but not much longer, especially if there was a series of journeys to be taken over a period of time. For one period of three weeks we took buses every other day – I didn't relish the idea of not going to the toilet ever again!

'Sometimes I felt very panicky on the buses – I would always try to sit next to a window that would open and to keep my face and neck cool with water, do deep breathing, look out of the window and listen to mellow songs on the Walkman to calm down and distract myself from what once would have been the worse nightmare imaginable.

'One aspect that really helped was that everyone really did get diarrhoea so I wasn't alone. All the travellers we met would talk about their bowel habits just after meeting them. Suddenly diarrhoea was not a taboo subject – the whole world understood if anyone had to disappear in mid-sentence to find a toilet. Even a nasty accident was not uncommon among "normal" people and was treated with sympathy and humour.

'I firmly believe, after my experiences, that it is important to face up to whatever the worst fears are – little by little. Being able to cope with them gives new confidence to push yourself further. It wasn't very long ago that I had to break a forty minute Underground journey to go to the toilet on many occasions. Before that there was a time when I couldn't leave the house for more than half an hour without panicking. Now I've just had the best year ever, something which would have been unimaginable a couple of years ago. I hope this will give some of you hope because things can get better. My problems haven't left me but I feel I am running my life now and it is not my bowels that are making the rules.'

Martin's tale is as follows:

'My first experience with IBS, as far as I can remember, was about seventeen years ago, while having my hair cut. I vividly remember the nauseous feeling and panic that set in. I was sure I was going to be sick. All I could do was to suddenly remember an urgent appointment as an excuse to get out and rush home to the toilet. I wasn't sick but the pain and spasms frightened me. I didn't dwell on it, until it happened again on the train on the way to work.

'I visited my GP who prescribed liquorice tablets. And later, I had my first barium meal.

'Things seemed to settle down and it was couple of years later that my tummy decided to rebel. I had been promoted at work and had moved to London. It was wonderful. I had a whole new life, new friends, my own flat. Although I was used to travelling everywhere on the tube, one day I suddenly felt that feeling, my tummy turned, I became drenched in sweat and I needed the toilet. I was desperately gasping for air, not knowing whether I was going to die, have a heart attack, be sick or have diarrhoea! After leaping off at the next station I calmed myself down and very shakily returned home.

'I was alternating between constipation and diarrhoea, and the frequency of my attacks was increasing. I was walking four miles to work to avoid tubes, and long journeys were a nightmare. I was told that I was suffering from anxiety. I was then put on tranquillizers – for the next four years! I remember very little, except that my world had got smaller and I was, by this time, being treated for agoraphobia. I had three weeks off work, sitting on the floor for days on end, until I snapped. I realized that only I could help myself. I felt that the psychiatrists were more stupid that I was. I knew I was sensible, but had become out of control through drugs and unfortunately alcohol, which was the only thing that could relieve my depression, temporarily, but only made things worse the next day. I screamed (inwardly, fortunately for my neighbours!) and sat by the toilet throwing all the hundreds – I mean hundreds – of tranquillizers away that I had been prescribed, which I had accumulated by cleverly ordering repeat prescriptions very regularly.

'Learning to cope with IBS was not easy, but some time later I discovered the IBS Network, put everything into perspective and started to take control of my life. I do have a medical condition. It is IBS. It comes and goes. I am not mentally unstable, although I have "learned" symptoms of agoraphobia and did have panic attacks, anxiety and depression brought on by the medical profession's lack of knowledge and understanding. The anti-depressants helped both ways, especially with the sedative side, allowing me to be rational in awkward situations.

'Several trips to the toilet, plenty of water and other fluids, and keeping very busy doing things around the house and garden are my way of coping. It is fatal to sit down, mope and get depressed – put on a favourite happy record and dance around the house until tomorrow, when you know you'll be OK again – until the next time!'

Coping with IBS long-term

IBS is rarely a short-lived problem and, although some people do recover from it, you may reach a point where you need to adjust to the realization that it isn't going to go away easily.

Judith Brice is a psychiatrist who has struggled with IBS herself. She says that people with chronic intestinal illnesses have to cope with psychological aspects that often go unacknowledged.[3] You may feel the loss of the healthy person you once were. Your self-image may change, and there may be a feeling that the illness is somehow your fault. People who suffer from IBS also have to live with the unpredictability it brings – they don't always know when the symptoms will occur.

Dr Brice says, 'A certain amount of predictability is vital for planning and controlling one's life. When you can't plan from one month to the next, or even from one week to the next, because you can't say how your health will be, that unreliability tends to eat away at your mood, your psyche, your self-esteem, and finally at the very relationships that have the power to make you feel good about your life.'

We also have to cope with embarrassing and 'socially unacceptable' symptoms. Frightening symptoms, confusing symptoms, too. Dr Brice says that good care of oneself doesn't guarantee that the condition will go away and there is often confusing advice about what constitutes good self-care so that sufferers find themselves on an endless search for the best way to handle the symptoms.

Because IBS often has a psychosomatic label attached, there is also the implication from some quarters that intestinal illness is caused by the sufferers themselves because of their lack of control over their emotional state. Sufferers often feel guilty, or may be made to feel guilty, that they are somehow less emotionally mature than others because they cannot handle the stresses of daily life without becoming ill. If your self-esteem is low anyway because of the condition, self-blame can only worsen it. As Dr Brice says, 'Don't let anyone convince you that the solution lies solely with you and your willpower.'

Nearest and dearest

Support from family and friends can make all the difference to how we are able to cope. Here is what some sufferers say on the subject. Tricia, who told her story earlier, writes:

'I think it's terribly important to get the support of your family and friends. Their attitude can make or break you. My partner of 10 years is only now beginning to appreciate that I have a problem, thanks mainly to wider public awareness. At first he would get really angry with me if we were out in the car and I asked to stop so I could go to the loo. I think he felt I was being terribly weak and pathetic and imagining everything, and he couldn't understand how a normally sane person turned into a gibbering wreck because she wanted to go to the loo. Eventually, anticipating his reaction, I found I was dashing to the loo umpteen times before we even got in the car. In contrast, my mother knew exactly how I felt and was terribly patient with me and never complained no matter how many times we had to stop; I found I never needed to go so often when I was with her. Books on IBS, left open at strategic places, seemed to convince my partner that I wasn't subnormal and that there were other people in the world who had the same crippling problem, and he is now more tolerant.'

Some people don't feel able to talk to relatives and friends about their suffering at all. Daisy says:

'I have not told anyone, even the man I've lived with for 15 years. I grit my teeth and pray. I feel *stupid* for being so oversensitive and overreactive.'

Natalie is lucky in that although none of her immediate friends have IBS she has plenty of helpful support from them. She says:

'Some friends have helped with the practical things like taking the children to school on the (fortunately rare) mornings that I can't escape from the bathroom for more than 60 seconds. Others have provided newspaper articles related to the problem or recommended books, and as a result I've learnt quite a lot about IBS.'

'I sometimes marvel that I've still got a husband and a son, it's been so bad for them. They should have permanent halos above their heads, as they make every allowance possible and support me through every gut-churning episode. It has been known for my son to be sitting outside the toilet door, talking me through the pain, rather than let me suffer alone,' says Victoria.

Try to make sure you have people around who are sympathetic and will offer you practical and emotional support when you need it. Research has shown that 'social support' can have a positive impact on not only mental health but physical health as well. Social support can include the support of partner, family and friends, as well as membership of self-help groups.

Why does such support help? Researchers say it is because it can bring about changes in behaviour.[4] For instance, people in self-help groups can be encouraged to make changes in their lifestyle which will promote improved health. Emotional support provided during stressful episodes may reduce the severity of the illness, as well as helping the sufferer to cope better and even recover.

Psychological factors are at work in the benefits offered by social support. For instance, stress can lead to lowered self-esteem, which can in turn lead to depression and increased susceptibility to disease. On the other hand, the knowledge that support is there if a sufferer needs it can increase self-esteem and give a sense of personal control, both of which are related to successful coping. Social support gives sufferers greater resilience in the face of adversity.

Health care workers can provide information and advice. Friends and relatives can assist in practical ways by giving the sufferer lifts, or helping with other chores.

Non-supportive relationships can have a bad effect on a patient's well-being. In another study, depressed rheumatoid arthritis patients who reported minimal support and bad relationships experienced the highest level of symptoms.[5] Close relationships can serve as a potential source of stress as well as a source of support for individuals coping with chronic illness. Ill-health is more pronounced for those who lack support.

Judy says:

'Lots of people haven't heard of IBS and don't know how much it affects your life. Most of my friends and relatives haven't the faintest idea what IBS is and even though I have described my symptoms, because it's not life-threatening or even something well known, I feel they don't really think there's anything the matter.

'If we had visual signs like a broken leg we would get much more sympathy from those around us, instead of the same old phrase, "Oh, not another bad stomach. It must be something you've eaten." If only it was that simple.'

Try to surround yourself with people who are able and willing to help you. If you don't get the support you need from your family, look outside it to friends or perhaps a self-help group.

Self-help groups

Self-help groups can be a good source of social support. Maisie writes:

'Self-help groups can have advantages and disadvantages. It can be very disheartening to discover that some people have been suffering from IBS for up to 20 years, but they can reassure you that you are not suffering alone, they can provide an outlet to vent your emotions and to gain a sympathetic ear or two and they are a way of exchanging ideas on how to help each other. Talking about bowels all evening can be very amusing and is sure to give you a damn good bellyache. After all, laughter is the best medicine.'

All the people to whom we have talked about IBS self-help groups have said much the same thing: that they discussed their symptoms and how they had been in the time since they last met, as well as particular issues of concern to IBS sufferers and treatments that have been found helpful. Most groups have occasional speakers – gastroenterologists, aromatherapists, dieticians and homeopaths, for example. The size of the groups varies from five people to as many as thirty-seven, although most groups seem to contain a core of about eight people.

Here are some people's experiences of how self-help groups have helped them.

'I find the self-help group interesting: it's good to know how others have suffered and sometimes found solutions. I feel the group is supportive. I live alone – fortunately, as my symptoms are very anti-social. I haven't any other support – my employers are not sympathetic, and neither is the doctor. Friends don't understand.'

'I decided to join a group just to have someone to talk to who understands what I am going through – it helps knowing my fellow sufferers. I can count on my friends to be sympathetic, and my employers, but I'm afraid my doctor isn't really concerned.'

'I joined to get more information about IBS and to listen to other sufferers' problems and see whether any treatments have been of help to them. I think on the whole I have had quite a lot of help in understanding how other people have dealt with the complaint. At the group we are treated with understanding and know that everything is done in confidence. All the members are friendly and cooperative. I can't count on anyone else for support – so many people seem unaware of the problem and are not all that interested in something that does not affect them. The doctor has not discussed this with me either.'

It can be seen that meeting other IBS sufferers can provide a source of support which is missing from other relationships. So many sufferers feel that they cannot discuss their IBS problems with their partners and colleagues, and being able to relax and talk to others who understand can be a great boost. The majority of people who wrote to us found self-help groups beneficial, although a few were sceptical:

'The doctors couldn't help me so I felt I was on my own and had to help myself. The only way I could think of was to talk to other people with IBS to see if we could establish what causes it and how we can get better. I've been five times, but it hasn't helped me at all. It has just rubbed in how hopeless it all is. The sort of people who attend are desperate, so it is one desperate person trying to help another. It didn't make me feel any better knowing that most people in the group had had it for 10 to 15 years and I had a long way to go. Unfortunately, nobody has the same symptoms as me so I might as well be sitting in the same room with someone suffering from another illness. We all want a doctor with IBS to attend! Some of my friends and colleagues are sympathetic to my IBS, and that's one reason I don't feel desperate to talk to people in a self-help group. With all the good will in the world, no one can really understand what I am going through. I don't know anyone who has my symptoms and who is in dreadful pain every single minute of the day, and has been for the last three years. If there is someone out there then I'd like to have a very long chat with them, please!'

Lifting the taboo

'IBS and its symptoms are thought to be funny or "not quite nice" by many people, so we have to suffer silently and attempt to feel like attractive, acceptable human beings in spite of it.' (Glenda)

There needs to be a change in attitude in the general public. Half of the people taking part in our survey said that they didn't know anyone else with IBS and a further 25 per cent knew only one other person. This makes it something that often has to be coped with alone in spite of it affecting such a large percentage of the population. Even if you do know someone else who has been diagnosed as having IBS they may have completely different symptoms and cope quite differently.

Although IBS is so common, there is a taboo, certainly in our society, about anything to do with bowel functions. They are supposed to be private and personal and the message is – keep it to yourself! This taboo can lead to problems for the individual sufferer. Not only can she or he remain isolated and lonely (quite unnecessarily so, given the prevalence of IBS) but she or he may feel unable to tell her or his family or even doctor about it, so support and treatment will not be forthcoming. A large number of people with IBS do not talk about it at all to anyone except perhaps close family members, and nearly half the people in our survey talked to no one at all. It is quite possible you know several people who also suffer but if every one thinks they shouldn't mention it everyone will continue to be isolated.

Nicky, a 31-year-old single mother, says:

'I think it would be better if things like IBS could be talked about more openly, and that it wasn't such a taboo subject because it involves a normal bodily function such as going to the toilet.'

Hattie, who has had IBS for nine years, says:

'I talk to people now about it but it was the biggest hurdle to be able to admit that I had such a personal problem.'

Coping through diet

As IBS is a condition affecting the gut, a common way of coping is regulating what you eat. Judy, a 31-year-old who has had the condition for 10 years and suffers from pain, constipation, bloating and wind, says:

'I find that if I keep my meals small the symptoms aren't so bad. I don't go out for meals.'

One sufferer, Malcolm, a bus driver, says:

'I only have one small meal a day, in the evening, and the symptoms have improved.'

Madeleine recommends:

'The best thing probably is to eat little and often, never to go too long without food and to eat a small, nourishing breakfast (which I don't always do) and certainly to avoid eating late in the evening, particularly anything strong or indigestible.'

Siobhan has found that foods containing vinegar, tomato sauce, chutneys, pickled beetroot, meat pastes, wine etc. or acid oranges and lemons as well as bran and stodgy foods don't suit her.

Some have found help simply through giving up tea and coffee, alcohol, citrus fruits, fatty foods, wheat or milk. Others have to stick to rigid diets. A wide range of diets may help IBS, but they are often extremely restrictive, expensive and time-consuming.

'For the last three and a half years I have based my diet on the Hay System as described by Doris Grant and Jean Joice in their very readable book, *Food Combining For Health*,' says Fran. 'The basic principle is that one should not eat protein and starch foods at the same meal, but you will have to read the book to understand that better. Because I also cook for a growing family and have a full social life I do not follow it strictly, but enough to have cut out most of the pain, the exhaustion of "illness", the constipation, heartburn, sleeplessness and build-up of tooth plaque! If I could only follow this fairly difficult regime perfectly, maybe it would be even better!

'Then I cut down on sugar, milk and wheat products. This cut out all the nausea and, provided I don't eat wheat products after tea-time, the nocturnal churning of the stomach.

'Finally, I take a personal homeopathic remedy, which sends me to sleep in the event of over-indulgence in alcohol or a churning stomach caused by after-hours wheat intake or just plain overeating late in the evening.'

It is important to weigh up the pros and cons of restrictive diets. If one works for you it may offer great relief from your symptoms and therefore be of value. On the other hand, you might feel your life is limited enough already! This is how Zoe feels about giving up wheat:

'I don't think the improvement sufficient to give up wheat totally. Besides, I'm sure it would be near impossible, as bread forms the major part of my diet. IBS has deprived me of so many of the things in life which I used to enjoy doing that to have to give up something which I like eating and gives me pleasure is a depressing prospect!'

Not everyone finds a 'healthy' diet helps. For Pat, it's just the opposite:

'This sounds very unhealthy, but I'm OK with crisps, packet food, sweets, meat, nothing green, no pulses, cabbage, spicy foods. "Natural" food seems to be worse for me.'

Cindy attended a clinic specializing in detecting food intolerances.

'I attended the clinic a few years ago and followed the exclusion diet. It was through this that I discovered I have an intolerance to milk and dairy products. They are really helpful and supportive there and I did feel that at last someone was trying to help. My doctor at that time insisted that it was "nerves" and that I was a bored housewife who needed to find something to occupy her mind and stop worrying about her stomach.'

Food intolerance does have significant implications for IBS sufferers and is discussed in more detail in Chapter 6.

Other tips

'At present I am taking concentrated slippery elm capsules, and did feel a soothing of my stomach at first, with less wind, but reverted to the usual condition after a few days. This happened to me with linseed oil – initial improvement only.'

'Slippery elm is very helpful internally where inflammatory irritation exists as diarrhoea, dysentery etc. You can buy slippery elm powder from a herbalist – the health stores mainly sell a commercial drink called slippery elm but containing other ingredients, though they also sell slippery elm tablets if the drink proves unpalatable.'

Ursula has had IBS for over 30 years:

'However, before Christmas I went into my health store and got two lots of tablets – peppermint oil tablets and New Era Combination E Tissue Salts – and I am pleased to be able to tell you I have been much better and feel I am more able to cope.'

Others have tried a wide variety of remedies:

'For years I was on codeine phosphate until I changed to a new doctor who took me off them and has since been trying various prescriptions. I have a permanent one for loperamide capsules, which I take if travelling or on an outing. My doctor advised me to use them only as a back-up for confidence, as did the hospital specialist.'

'At present I am trying Colpermin capsules, which are peppermint. They are definitely helping with the bloated feeling.'

'I have found that mashed potato often calms the seething turbulence within. It doesn't always work but sometimes has a soothing effect on both wind and pain.'

'I have tried an elimination diet and found I was much better giving up red meats, rich foods, jams and, strangely, vinegar.'

'Walking after meals helps to reduce gas.'

'Since I stopped drinking cow's milk about six months ago I believe my IBS has improved considerably. I read about lactose intolerance and decided to give it a whirl, on the "nothing ventured, nothing gained" principle, known only too well by IBS folk.'

'The most beneficial thing I have found is yoga taught with relaxation. It is excellent and I combine my lessons with a daily workout at home.'

'My problems began seven years ago after a holiday in Kenya. Things have definitely improved over the years but I can still remember with clarity the times when I didn't quite make it to the loo in time. I now never go anywhere without my "shit kit"' – a small cosmetic bag with wet wipes, toilet paper, clean panties and a plastic bag and also my codeine phosphate. Just knowing I carry those items with me gives me peace of mind and makes me feel calmer.'

'After two years of diarrhoea, flatulence, nausea and losing two stone in weight and utter misery I thought, at 80 years of age, this is it. With the aid of an anti-spasmodic and codeine phosphate, also careful watch of diet, I feel so much better.'

'Some divine intervention led, for reasons not connected with IBS, to taking lecithin capsules and within three to four days the symptoms of IBS became considerably lessened and controllable. By taking three to four capsules daily I have found not a total cure but an amazing improvement in my condition.'

The range of things people with IBS try in order to help themselves is vast. Some people live constantly in the hope that this or that will be the cure at last. It can be very dispiriting when time and time again you are disappointed. In the 20 years that Susan Backhouse has had IBS she has tried traditional drugs, peppermint capsules, garlic capsules, slippery elm, a wide selection of herbs, Bach flower remedies, acupuncture, homeopathy, exclusion diets, dairy-free diets, gluten-free diets, high-fibre diets, giving up tea and coffee, eating lots of yogurt, relaxation, yoga – the list goes on. And she realizes she is not atypical.

'I know the hope and the disappointment when things are tried, but don't help. In fact, the best thing I have done is co-found the IBS Network with Christine, because suddenly there were letters from a great number of people with similar, and different, stories to mine. I found it easier to talk about my IBS and no longer felt anywhere near so isolated. My way of coping now is to work with others towards improving things for all of us who have IBS.'

Chapter 6

The Connection Between Lifestyle and IBS

'My IBS is affected by pressure at work, very little support and the lack of someone "there for me". I do get anxious and I'm not good at sharing my problems. I'm trying to rectify this.'

IBS affects a wide range of people living a wide range of lifestyles. It used to be thought that it was a specifically Western condition, but it is now known to occur in developing countries. Both men and women suffer from it. It is suffered by all age groups, and some people feel they have always had it. There is no typical kind of lifestyle that makes IBS more likely and there is no lifestyle formula that will guarantee an IBS-free existence. However, in this chapter we will look at the ways in which IBS sufferers have tried to improve their way of life through dealing with stress, adopting better eating habits and increasing exercise and consider if this has had a direct effect on their symptoms and their ability to cope with them.

Can stress cause or aggravate IBS?

The professionals tend to believe that stress plays a large part in IBS, and people with the condition are often advised to reduce the stress in their lives. But how easy is it to control stress?

It does not seem to be simply a matter of taking up meditation, learning relaxation techniques or even finding out what causes you stress and then removing it from your life. In our survey we found that many IBS sufferers have made changes to their lifestyle in order to reduce stress; some people have taken drastic measures such as taking early retirement, changing their job or getting divorced, only to find that although they are experiencing a lot less stress their IBS is no better.

We live in a world that causes us, at times, to suffer extreme stress and anxiety. It is often not possible to remove the source of stress from our lives, and it may not always be easy to deal with the stress in a way that doesn't do any harm to ourselves or others.

Stress is much discussed and written about these days. People were once said to be suffering from 'nerves' and with that there was an implication that they were weak and unable to cope with life. Now there seems to be some acknowledgement that stress is something we all have to deal with and that people cope in different ways.

When researchers study IBS patients they find that many say their symptoms are made worse by stress, and one study found that half their patients recalled an acute episode of stress before their first symptoms.[1] Sometimes the beginning of IBS can be traced back to a time of emotional turmoil such as a bereavement, an accident or an operation (although there is evidence that certain operations can cause physiological changes that give rise to IBS symptoms). This is, apparently, very common amongst diarrhoea-predominant IBS sufferers. Another study done in 1982 concluded that some people have a biological predisposition to respond to any stressful situation with increased movements in the colon.[2] In a large study of 800 IBS sufferers, it was found that stress affected their IBS in three-quarters of them, half of whom said that stress led to abdominal pain.[3]

A study done by gastroenterologists Kumar, Pfeffer and Wingate found that their IBS patients were more anxious and obsessive than other people, but not more depressive. Kumar and his colleagues say that the idea that IBS is primarily a psychopathological condition has been attractive to the medical profession because of the lack of evidence, up until recently, of something organically wrong. They say that some researchers suggest that it is a symptom of depression, others that IBS patients have a pain-prone personality and that pain represents a means of emotional expression! There are some who believe that IBS is a manifestation of 'illness behaviour'. Consequently, psychotherapy or anti-depressants have been advocated.

More recently, however, studies have indicated that IBS could be an organic disorder. What then, asked Kumar and his fellow researchers, of the anxiety associated with the condition? Could it be the consequence rather than the cause of IBS? And have the psychopathological aspects of IBS been over-emphasized, due to flaws in some of the studies? Comparing IBS sufferers with healthy controls might reveal more about the differences between the well and the unwell rather than IBS specifically, for instance. In their study they compared IBS sufferers with people suffering from benign organic gastrointestinal disorders such as duodenal ulcer, gallstones and inflammatory bowel disease as well as with healthy people. They found that the IBS patients were more anxious and obsessional than healthy people but there was no difference for depression or phobic tendencies. Those suffering from the other gastrointestinal disorders were in between the other two groups. They say that these results are, 'consistent with the state of mind of a patient who is still searching for some rational explanation – and some effective therapy – for his or her symptoms' and that 'IBS patients are not helped by being told that "there's nothing wrong", when this is manifestly at odds with their own experience'.

They go on to say that when effective treatment is found, it is likely that there will be no greater levels of anxiety and other neuroses than you would expect in any group of people suffering from a chronic gastrointestinal disorder.

Is stress responsible for *your* IBS?

'If I hear the word STRESS again from my doctor I shall scream.'

When IBS sufferers are told their condition is due to stress, it can be very frustrating and can seem too simplistic.

'Stress makes me dash to the loo more, but I still have problems on calm days.'

'Severe symptoms can often occur even when my life is going well.'

'If I have symptoms due to stress, they tend to be mild and easy to cope with by comparison with other times. Stress will aggravate a problem if it's already there, i.e. if I feel queasy anyway and then get upset, it tends to get worse. But stress is not the cause – the symptoms are too severe and the stress too little. The most stressful thing in my life is constant nausea and continual pain, everything else seems to pale in comparison,'

says Andrea, and her feelings that it is IBS that causes the stress in her life are echoed by many:

'I honestly feel that the only stress I have difficulty coping with is my painful gut, which adversely affects the quality of my life far more than the cancer which I have lived with for the past number of years.'

'Many people who are suffering from diarrhoea for just a few days are very stressed and fed up – so people like us are going to be very stressed as the condition lasts for so long and it is too embarrassing to discuss with others.'

'The anxiousness over IBS symptoms causes stress, which worsens the symptoms, hence creating a vicious circle.'

The contradictions experienced by many of us are voiced by Maxine:

'For myself, I have yet to understand if stress can be such a large part of suffering with IBS. Over the past few years I have had traumas: buying a house, becoming a single parent, money worries, housing worries, etc., and yet I can say that IBS never presented itself, unless IBS triggers quite some time after the events.'

Mo also feels there is no straightforward answer to the IBS and stress dilemma.

'The past few years have been difficult ones for a number of reasons, so it would be easy to put the symptoms down to this. But I am not satisfied that this is the only reason. I have had plenty of other stressful incidents in the past, and have not suffered in this way. Equally, I have been on holiday and enjoying myself, and still had the symptoms. The trouble is, if no true cause is known, then if you are not careful you can get paranoid about food and become stressed about the possible stress!'

Annette says:

'The usual answer from the medical profession is stress. This suggests my problem is psychosomatic not biological. I firmly believe it is the latter, and doctors haven't got the answer so stress is a good word to pacify patients.

'One of my worst bouts last year was walking over Welsh hills with my family – about 10 of us, aged between 2 and 80. A happy band, enjoying the walk. We were coming back and wham! it was that familiar gut problem. I asked my son for his house keys and ran like hell, shouting, 'Don't follow me!' But I didn't make it. Luckily, I was washed and changed before they arrived home.'

It is not uncommon to find that IBS strikes when we at last have a chance to relax and enjoy ourselves.

Sean doesn't feel he has much stress in his life.

'My doctor seems to favour the stress theory, and talks of "taking it more easy", "getting away from it all", and what he cryptically refers to as "taking the edge off things". Of course, I realize that stress is a relative term and that all of us have some stress in our lives; and while I definitely belong to the "nervy and fastidious" brigade, rather than the "laid back and easy-going", I can't pretend that I have a huge amount of stress in my life.'

There are some who feel stress is not a factor in their IBS. Ruby is one:

'I have not been able to identify stress as a cause of aggravation of my condition. As I now have little stress, almost none at all really, I cannot include it as something which affects my IBS.'

And Maisie agrees:

'In my opinion, stress had nothing to do with my onset of IBS. I get very angry when anyone suggests otherwise. I was off work for seven months solely to concentrate on me – to get better – but it didn't work. I got worse.'

In spite of this, over 70 per cent of those taking part in our study said that stress aggravated their IBS. For Hazel, stress is a direct trigger of her symptoms. She says:

'I'm sure stress makes my IBS much worse. I'm rather a perfection-ist and get very strung up if things don't go the way they should.'

Fiona, having made significant changes in the food she eats, found that this has helped her symptoms:

112

'It seems to be something that I can exert a positive control over, unlike stress, with which I still find myself constantly battling. Any stress attack brings on the symptoms. I become stressful with myself when I don't achieve the high standards I set and I also worry about events before they happen. My symptoms have decreased over the last few months. I think that if I were calmer as a person they may even disappear totally.'

And for Lucy, the relationship between stress and IBS is very closely linked:

"The difference between me and people without IBS is that I find certain things stressful or anxiety-causing that a 'normal' person wouldn't. I feel anxious about the possibility of having to go to the toilet too frequently (I don't care how often I have to have a wee – weird!) or having to have a crap at a time of day or a place where no one else would (e.g. a party, someone's house for dinner, etc.). It does take away the anxiety a bit if I'm with people who are open about bowel habits. For some reason I can't admit to having IBS symptoms when a "normal" person would admit to getting the shits before an interview, exam, scary meeting etc. Because I feel stressed because I have IBS it's impossible to tell whether I caused the IBS by handling the stress badly or whether I am more stressed because of IBS. What came first, the stress or the IBS?'

When we asked people with IBS what they thought the cause was, several cited reasons such as stressful jobs, family problems, being involved in an accident, bereavement, depression and general stress and worry. It is known that specific hormonal changes can occur when a person is under stress and that they in turn can affect the bowels. In a discussion on IBS and stress Dr Heaton says, 'There have been some remarkable experiments on the effects of stress on sigmoid colon motility. The point which came out was that it was not the pain inflicted on the volunteers that caused the sigmoid colon to become active but the hostile reaction when the volunteers decided that they could not tolerate it any more.'[5]

This has interesting implications for sufferers of pain: it means that it may be possible to reduce colonic activity by using pain-control techniques. (See Chapter 5 for more on pain control.)

Does personality make a difference?

In our study we found that a high proportion of sufferers described themselves as 'worriers'. Is this the cause of their IBS, or does living with the condition turn them into anxious people? Worrying about IBS will very likely make it worse.

Lucy feels she generally worries more than other people might, although most of what she worries about is related to IBS.

'I find it hard to stop thinking about something that has annoyed me. I tend to brood on things and keep coming back to them even though I try not to. I worry about some things happening that might never occur, for example running out of petrol or breaking down on the motorway. This way of thinking applies to IBS-related worries as well – I constantly worry about "what if something happens" rather than solving the problem when it arises.

'Because I have IBS I spend a lot of time worrying about whether or not it will affect me during each day. Whenever there is anything major to worry about I will spend a lot of time going over and over the possibilities in my mind. I have been told that I always need something to worry about – as if I enjoy it!

'Having said this, no one other than my boyfriend would ever know I was worrying. Everyone else believes I'm incredibly calm and unruffled by life. I think this calm exterior can be dangerous and means that there is a lot of suppressed anxiety which I believe manifests itself in IBS.'

We asked people if they thought that aspects of their character made IBS more difficult to deal with. Common themes were setting very high standards for oneself, having difficulty relaxing, caring too much what people think, finding it difficult to talk about IBS, insecurity and lack of confidence and self-esteem.

Not surprisingly, it was clear that our sample of sufferers had a wide range of personalities, lifestyles and ways of coping with IBS and life in general. Living with pain and the other symptoms for any length of time can certainly cause a person to change their behaviour, and even, say some, their personality.

'It has made me less confident, more introverted, less tolerant, more impatient.'

'My personality, that's changed dramatically. I'm nasty, vicious and aggressive and can't tolerate much of anything.'

What causes stress?

There are some things that most people would find stressful – an important relationship going wrong, harassment or victimization, financial problems, homelessness, for example. It is believed that change can cause stress, even change for the better. Stress is also caused by feeling out of control. However, it can be a very individual thing. The list of stressful life events has divorce as highly stressful, but if the divorce is wanted then it could mean that a person's worry and anxiety levels are reduced.[6] A lifestyle that to one person is peaceful and relaxing can be very boring for the next person – and even boredom is stressful.

Here are some explanations of what causes some sufferers stress, starting with Lucy, who works as a graphic designer:

'I feel stressful if I have to do things I don't feel comfortable doing – things which I know will cause my IBS to get worse, for example travelling with people I don't know well (or who don't know I've got IBS), working on location, where I can't go to the toilet inconspicuously, eating with people I don't feel comfortable with, travelling somewhere just after eating (the list goes on!).'

'The things that cause me stress include early morning appointments, going to church in the morning, being invited out for meals or to stay with anybody at their home.'

'I suffer stress if I feel under constant pressure at work and also if I am underemployed. Other people's tantrums and distress upset me. Stress builds up if I am subjected to incessant noise.'

'I think any stress was due to isolation on account of my husband's 24-hour-a-day job (as a doctor) and no extended family.'

'My husband being in the army and him going away a lot.'

'I live in a neighbourhood where there is a lot of vandalism, glue sniffing and young people forever tormenting older people. Life today causes stress unless you are someone who doesn't care.'

'Meeting deadlines on VDU work.'

'Being a single parent to three children, low pay, an ageing parent, harassment at work, threats of job loss through cuts recession, loneliness because not in a relationship at present.'

'Tubes, crowded transport, car travel in the morning. Awkward people. Crowds pushing and shoving, being squashed in a crowd. Not being treated fairly at work, too much work, too little time to do it and boss being unreasonable.'

'People saying nasty things or my boss on my back for any reason, or a heavy work load. I panic.'

'I worry over work, not fulfilling my potential, money problems, not knowing how to use my talents and fighting fatigue.'

In addition, family and relations were frequently cited in our study as the cause of stress.

How stress affects us

Dorothy explains what happens when she is under stress and how it aggravates her IBS:

'Under stress I tend to neglect my own needs. I also get very angry that I seem unable to switch off and put myself first. When stressed I breathe shallowly, never seem to relax, have disordered eating (binge eating), all of which worsens my IBS. I feel stressed when I feel powerless to change any part of my life, e.g. work, accommodation. I freeze in response to any threat or change (real or perceived) rather than act/try something/ask for help or advice. I isolate myself in a sort of psychological straitjacket.'

And Susie, who is 42 and has had the condition for over seven years, describes the link for her between IBS and stress:

'Knowing I have to go out, e.g. for an appointment, causes me stress because of the agoraphobia I suffer from. This causes me to go to the toilet frequently, up to 9 or 10 times in the previous 18 to 24 hours. The pain caused by wind can also be worse. Fear of disapproval and rejection is probably the major factor in my agoraphobia and the feeling that my body will let me down by diarrhoea or nausea increases the stress.'

When sufferers experience traumas the way they relate to their IBS can alter, as Lucy describes:

'Important life-changing events (e.g. the breakdown of a relationship) have made my IBS much worse and the feeling of anxiety is raised to the forefront of my consciousness. Because of this it has been easier to talk about the anxiety and express it, come to terms with it and cope with it. Probably because it is socially acceptable to feel anxious, get stomach cramps, feel nauseous and have diarrhoea during a major trauma like this, it is possible to admit to these feelings and be comforted by friends. Other than a major trauma bringing on these symptoms I would never let anyone know about IBS symptoms normally.'

Panic

Sixty per cent of the people taking part in our study said they had experienced panic attacks at some time. There is a specifically named condition called panic disorder and one American study tried to find out if people with IBS symptoms were really suffering from this problem.[7] People who had IBS symptoms and experienced panic attacks were treated with anti-panic medication. The results were a quick improvement in their gastrointestinal symptoms. It concluded that there are strong links between gastrointestinal complaints and panic disorder.

The authors of the study considered it worth mentioning if the subject's family had a history of agoraphobia, depression, alcoholism and so on but there was no mention of how the symptoms might be caused by non-genetic factors, such as the subject being under a lot of pressure. It would also be interesting to know whether the improvement continued once medication had been stopped.

What do we do about stress?

Many of those who feel that stress is significant to their IBS realize that they need to make changes in their lives but often feel unable to do do. May is 60, a housewife, and has had IBS for eight years.

'I think my stress is caused by loneliness. I have three lovely daughters who are marvellous to me, they help me in all sorts of ways, but they have their own lives to lead. I need to change my life, but I don't know how.'

Anita is 21, and explains:

'I suffer stress from the inability to do things I'm fully capable of, physically and mentally. Living with parents is a major problem, but I can't afford to move out. I also suffer from situations I want to change but can't from low self-esteem.'

Even getting out of the stressful situation doesn't necessarily result in instant recovery. Frances is 40. She was married to an alcoholic who was violent and is now trying to rebuild her life with another partner. She still suffers from the stress she endured during her marriage.

Hannah's main cause of distress is wind and the embarrassment is turning her into a hermit. It has been developing over the last 12 years.

'My life is very curtailed by this condition which is a great pity as after a very stressful life I have now reached much calmer waters. It seems very perverse that I coped with the stress and then I develop this stressful condition when my life has become so much freer as I now happily live on my own in a lovely area surrounded by kind and friendly people.'

Hannah is 70 and her general health is very good. She feels she could live a much fuller and outgoing life were it not for her condition. She goes on to say:

'If I did not fret so much about the possibility of being embarrassed or maybe embarrassing others by my wind problem, maybe it would not be such a problem.'

Coping with stress is fraught with contradictions, as Holly writes:

'It is right when they say avoid things that really upset you, but you can't hide forever.'

Ruby feels she has done a lot to try to improve her lifestyle but to no avail.

'I have tried to change my way of life by taking more exercise and changing my diet, but my life is probably as stress-free as it could possibly be. I have been unable to find the trigger which sets off the intense pain I suffer.'

Ruth has found practical ways to deal with stress:

'I have developed various ways to minimize the detrimental effect of stress. Vitamin supplements, especially B vitamins (which are yeast/sugar/lactose free as I am on an anti-candida diet), help but it has been very difficult when all the GP can do is say "it's your nerves" and push anti-depressants at you. These do not help the fatigue/depression or the constipation.'

The two ways of dealing with stress are to change your exposure or your mental response to it. If you feel your IBS is caused or aggravated by the tension and pressure in your life you may decide to take a long, fresh look at your situation and your attitudes.

Like pain, signs of stress are warnings to be heeded. Be aware of how you, as an individual, respond to pressure, frustration and feelings of impotence or guilt. Do you find it difficult to let go and to express emotions, whether happiness, fear, anger, sadness? Emotions kept inside often resort to a churning stomach. Have you tried eating when you're upset? Your body rebels against you 'swallowing your anger' down with your potatoes. You soon end up with stomach ache.

Imagine this scene: you are out with some friends. It's a lovely day and you are enjoying yourself. Then into your mind comes the thought – there isn't a toilet nearby, what if I need to go? And in no time, your body starts working and you do need to go – and quick! The feeling may pass, or it may not. At best, it's on your mind and clouds your enjoyment of the day. At worst, you feel panicky and overwhelmed.

Does it sound familiar to some of you? If it has happened to you you will be aware of the power of your mind and how your imagination can work against you.

It is also worth remembering that this power can be used for your benefit. It is very hard, though, to change your mindset and you need to work at it. Try not to always expect and fear the worst: concentrate on visualizing a pleasant or successful outcome instead of your feared one. When you wake up in the morning, and throughout the day when you remember, say positive affirmations to yourself. For instance:

- Today I feel calm and peaceful.
- I will feel good about my body and in control.
- My stomach feels warm and relaxed.
- I am in harmony with my body.
- Today I feel strong and capable.
- I have nothing to fear but my fear.

Dr Vernon Coleman, in his book *Bodypower*, writes of the value of daydreaming to relax the mind from tensions and pressures.[8]

He suggests focusing on a happy memory – a holiday, a beautiful place you've been to, for instance – and transporting yourself there. If you picture the place vividly you will be able to involve all your senses – smelling, hearing, feeling, tasting even, as well as seeing your surroundings. Keep the action peaceful and calm. You may want to lie down to daydream at first, especially if it is a long time since you have done it. With practice, however, you will be able to do it anywhere, anytime. Use it to escape to your own private, calm place when you need to. Many of us have been brought up to think that daydreaming is undesirable; parents and teachers often stop children from doing it. But Dr Coleman believes it has benefits over meditation. With the latter, the mind is cleared of all images and you concentrate on emptiness or perhaps one image. Daydreaming focuses on a loving, happy memory and will fill the daydreamer with loving, happy feelings. Daydreaming is, he says, a natural process whereby the mind can 'cut out' for our own protection.

Treating IBS and stress

In 1990 a study was completed by Dr Steve Wilkinson and Dr Nicky Rumsey, consultant gastroenterologist and research psychologist respectively at the Gloucester Royal Hospital.[9] It compared conventional drug treatment of severe IBS with a programme of six 90-minute sessions designed to teach groups of six to eight patients stress management and relaxation techniques. In this psychological programme a typical session would comprise a 15-minute talk, followed by a discussion and coffee. A second talk would be followed by a relaxation session and a summary. Topics covered were:

- What is IBS?
- The role of stress in IBS.
- Progressive muscle relaxation.
- Using relaxation constructively.
- Diet and fitness.
- Problem-solving.
- Long-term management of IBS.

The results of the study were encouraging. At the end of the treatment period, improvements in IBS symptoms and in measures of anxiety, depression and stress were evident for the majority of patients (26 out of a total of 37) whether they had received drug treatment or taken part in the psychological programme. However, six months after the end of the treatment period, patients in the psychological management group reported significantly fewer IBS symptoms and lower levels of anxiety, depression and stress than those patients who had received drug treatment.

The conclusion drawn was that group stress management is a viable, and even preferable, alternative to drugs for the treatment of IBS. When looking at why the treatment worked, the researchers say that they have to speculate but the patients clearly liked the approach. Some felt more in control of their condition, some were pleased with the information on how to deal with it and others felt their self-confidence had increased. Overall satisfaction was very high. (This may well be because of the general lack of support and information available to IBS sufferers until recently.)

The researchers report that this approach is much cheaper than conventional drug treatment. From August to October 1989 the 277 GPs who make up the Cleveland Family Practitioner Committee wrote nearly 6000 prescriptions for anti-spasmodics. This averaged out at seven prescriptions per GP per month, at a total cost of £34,062! Dr Rumsey believes that patients should be given an explanation of both the psychological and drug approach and allowed to choose which they would prefer.

It is to be hoped that the results of this study and of future research will encourage doctors and psychologists to consider setting up similar programmes on a more permanent basis. There is scope, too, for this kind of approach to be explored by self-help groups.

Other studies back up the findings of Drs Wilkinson and Rumsey. One found that when IBS patients were treated psychologically as opposed to medically and where anxiety levels were high beforehand, the anxiety decreased.[10] Psychological intervention alone was shown to reduce distress by the reduction of both anxiety and IBS symptoms.

Psychotherapy has also been used with success on patients in

Manchester. Dr Else Guthrie has found that specific techniques where the importance of the developing relationship between doctor and patient is a fundamental part of the treatment has helped many long-term sufferers.[11] Dr Guthrie reports a reduction in symptoms, less pain and a decrease in the limiting effect the bowel symptoms have on the sufferer's life. It seems that this method works well with people who believe that their pain is exacerbated by stress. Those who suffer constant pain don't seem to benefit. Those who have psychiatric symptoms such as anxiety and depression are likely to do well, according to Dr Guthrie.

Hypnotherapy can also be very effective in treating IBS where stress is a factor. At Dr Whorwell's clinic, also in Manchester, patients say that they can cope better with various other stresses in their lives by using the techniques learned during hypnosis. They are encouraged to see hypnotherapy as giving them a way to control their symptoms, rather than offering a magic cure. (See Chapter 3 for more on hypnotherapy.) Therapies such as massage and aromatherapy work well too. Because they are such relaxing and pleasurable experiences they have an indirect effect on the IBS symptoms, making them easier to cope with.

All complementary medicines have a holistic approach to treatment and therefore look at the patient's lifestyle and state of mind as well as physical symptoms.

Does exercise help IBS?

On the whole, our study found that although most people took regular exercise it wasn't felt to bring about a direct improvement in the symptoms. Some people are unable to exercise at all when having a bad patch. However, many agreed that it has a general uplifting effect.

Here are some sufferers' views on exercise:

'Exercise makes me feel worse physically, better mentally.'

'Good for settling the gut and improving mental outlook.' Brenda, who swims, does fitness sessions and hill walking.

'Swimming can help me pass trapped wind, or help to lessen the pain – or make it worse!'

'I have tried aerobics and keep fit – they seemed to aggravate IBS, in particular upper abdominal pain.'

'Intense physical activity, like cycling, gardening or even walking (I would no longer even attempt sports) tends to encourage attacks on subsequent days.'

'I cope mainly with the stress of IBS by playing tennis. It is very therapeutic whacking a tennis ball as hard as I can. It helps get rid of my frustration and gives me a sense of well-being. It's also great fun and laughter, after all, is the best medicine. The endorphins (natural painkillers) which the body produces during exercise also help. But the exercise has to be very vigorous and sustained to help me in any way. At least my tennis has improved!'

Diet

The connection between food and digestive function is an obvious one; many people with IBS feel that the food they eat has an effect on their symptoms, for better or worse. We found that two out of three people said that some foods aggravated them. Our study also showed that a high proportion of the sufferers taking part took great care with their food, many of them eating what is considered to be a healthy diet – low fat, little or no meat, plenty of fresh fruit and vegetables, unrefined carbohydrates. Many said they were eating these foods in order to help their IBS.

A change in diet is often one of the first steps IBS sufferers take, in the hope that it may ease or eradicate the symptoms. It is important to check with your doctor first before undertaking restrictive diets and, ideally, you should get the help of a dietician to ensure you get the required nutrients.

General dietary advice
It will almost certainly help you if you are able to follow the guidelines below:

- Eat a varied diet, full of food that you enjoy.
- Eat little and often – big meals are notoriously troublesome.
- Eat when relaxed, take your time and don't rush your meals. Consciously taste the food you eat. Listen to your body and stop eating when you have had enough.

123

- Eat when you feel hungry – not when the clock says it's time for food.
- Ensure a good intake of fruit and vegetables, especially green leafy ones which contain rich supplies of the vitamins and minerals that are most commonly found to be lacking in many ill or elderly people. A daily intake of raw or lightly cooked green vegetables or salad may also help protect against some of the more common and more serious diseases in Western society.
- Eat good-quality fresh food, preferably organic if this is available. The medical effects of insecticides and fertilizers sprayed on crops haven't been fully studied. Although organic fruit and vegetables are often expensive and hard to obtain, consumer demand may change this. More supermarkets are now providing organic produce. There is also a move towards the setting up of organic food co-ops modelled on the Seikatsu Club in Japan, where those joining pay a small amount each month and their groceries are delivered to the door each week. The co-ops are able to buy in bulk and buy direct from the suppliers, thus reducing the costs. They are especially beneficial to those living in rural areas.
- Fibre is important, especially if you suffer from constipation. However, do not rely on only one source of food for your fibre, for example wheat bran. Fibre is contained in beans, fruits (including dried fruit), vegetables, whole grains (such as oats, rice, barley, wheat and corn).
- Avoid highly processed food with additives and preservatives. Check the E numbers, as many of them are believed to cause digestive disturbances. (*Findout* lists all the E numbers and explains what their dangers are. [12])
- Stick to a diet that is generally low in fat but contains small amounts of good-quality, unrefined, cold-pressed oils such as sunflower, safflower or walnut oil (buy in small amounts and keep in the fridge because they can go rancid). There is no such thing as a completely cold-pressed oil because the pressing of the seed generates heat, but most commercial oils are pressed with extra heat. This may cause damage to the essential fatty acids, thus greatly

reducing the nutritional value of the oil. Refined oils are treated with a variety of chemicals, including bleach, deodorizer and petroleum-derived antioxidant. Olive oil is a good oil to cook with. In general, avoid frying as heat will destroy essential fatty acids. Avoid, as much as possible, hydrogenated and partially hydrogenated oils; the process of hydrogenation converts unsaturated fats into saturated fats in order to prolong shelf life.[13] In other words, a perfectly good oil like soya oil is turned into saturated fat which may clog up your arteries and interfere with your body's ability to use essential fatty acids.[14] If you regularly read the lists of ingredients on packets you will know it is very hard to find any processed food that doesn't contain these oils. From a health point of view, you are better eating small amounts of butter than normal amounts of margarine or low-fat spreads because of the hydrogenated oils they contain.

- Keep your intake of sugar, salt, caffeine and alcohol to a minimum.
- Avoid any foods you know don't agree with you. It may sound obvious, but it's worth mentioning.

High fibre or low fibre?

Doctors will often recommend that someone with IBS increase the fibre in their diet, no matter what the particular symptoms may be. In fact, if you suffer predominantly from diarrhoea, flatulence or bloating, a high-fibre diet can make things worse. One study found that pain and urgency to defecate were worsened significantly when coarse wheat bran was used.[15] Another problem is that some people simply put coarse wheat bran on their food and continue to eat a low-fibre diet otherwise. It is more advisable to increase the amount of fresh fruit and vegetables, particularly raw ones, and to eat unrefined, unprocessed food as much as possible. If this is very different from your usual diet, it should be done gradually to give your digestive system a chance to adjust.

There are two types of fibre: soluble (found in oats, pulses, bananas) and insoluble (found in wheat bran, cereal grains, apple and pear peel). Many people find that soluble fibre produces less bloating and is easier to digest than insoluble fibre.

Some people may find that a low-fibre diet suits them best. This means reducing or cutting out fruit and vegetables, nuts and wholegrain cereals, and the skin and gristle of meat. It allows fruit juices and includes highly refined products such as white flour. Such a diet may tend to be high in fat and sugar and is best worked out with the help of a dietician to ensure that you get all the nutrients you need.

High protein and low fat

One pair of researchers say that a diet low in fat and high in protein may help IBS.[16] Foods that fit that description include chicken and turkey without the skin, white fish, tofu and low-fat dairy products such as skimmed milk and low-fat cheeses.

Food intolerance

Some people with IBS find they cannot tolerate certain foods. Dairy products, wheat, citrus fruits and tea and coffee are common offenders. It may be worth cutting these out of your diet for a time to see if your symptoms improve and then reintroducing them one by one, every three days or so.

You may decide you want to try an exclusion diet to see if there are other foods that are aggravating you. The idea is that for a week or two you eat only two or three foods, preferably ones you rarely consume, and if your symptoms improve you can be pretty sure that food intolerance is your problem. Reintroduce other foods gradually and if all goes well you should notice your symptoms return soon after you eat an offending food. However, exclusion diets can be difficult and the results confusing; if they are done incorrectly they may result in multi-nutrient deficiencies, so it is important to undertake such a step with the guidance of a dietician. An added factor is the effect of additives and pesticides on the individual which can cause a reaction quite apart from an intolerance to the food itself.

Susan Backhouse went on two exclusion diets, carefully following advice from a book on the subject, but she wasn't sure if her symptoms improved during the exclusion period.

Then, after she began to reintroduce foods, she would find that one day wheat seemed fine but another day appeared to give her diarrhoea. In the end, she had to conclude that the results were inconclusive!

Ida has had bowel problems ever since she was a child. She eventually discovered that she cannot tolerate certain foods:

'I had always found that I was better without coffee or carrots in my diet but was convinced that something else in my diet was causing the problem. I went to a homeopathic doctor to have an allergy test. He diagnosed me as being sensitive to gluten, chocolate, monosodium glutamate and demerara sugar.

'This all happened five years ago and I have since followed this diet very carefully. I read every contents label in the supermarkets and am very aware of additives in our food. My friends and relations are all very understanding and we discuss the menu when I am visiting. I always take my own bread and my own gravy thickened with cornflour.

'I do still have the problem, but it is not nearly as bad as it was.'

We found that one person in seven is on a restricted diet because of their IBS. Below we look at some of these diets.

Wheat-free Wheat-free means, of course, cutting out wheat – no ordinary bread, pasta (although you can get pasta made out of buckwheat, which isn't wheat in spite of its name: read the ingredients to make sure it doesn't have extra wheat added), anything made out of wheat flour (watch out for things like soups for thickeners, some vending machine drinks, Ovaltine and Horlicks, baking powder and Mars bars, for example), no wheat bran or wheatgerm. Wheat can be found in some sausages, condiments, puddings, tinned foods, stuffing and many other foods. Avoid ingredients described as edible starch, modified starch, cereal filler, cereal binder and cereal protein.

Gluten-free diet No gluten means not eating wheat, barley, oats, and rye. Rice, maize and soya products are all gluten-free. You can't eat ordinary bread, but you can get gluten-free flour loaves, biscuits and cakes if you are able and willing to pay the earth! Rice cakes are a substitute for crackers, although they may take some getting used to (some say they taste of polystyrene). Cornflour, potato flour, rice flour, soya flour and arrowroot are gluten-free. Rice flour is great for cakes and biscuits; although it is hard to work with for pastry (it doesn't roll very easily), its nutty flavour is great for quiches. It is impossible to make pancakes with rice flour – try buckwheat flour instead. For thickening, use cornflour or potato flour. The latter is pretty awful in cakes, pastry and so on – the resulting product is like a stone. Fresh meats and bacon are gluten-free but many sausages are not. Most ready-made dishes have gluten in them, as do most cheap icecream, liquorice and many cheap confectionery items.

Starch-free diet A starch-free diet has been found by at least one sufferer to have helped her symptoms of distension and pain. This diet involves cutting out starch in all its forms including all grains, soya beans, potatoes and all cooked vegetables (starch is released in cooking but raw vegetables can be tolerated). The diet is then made up of fresh vegetables and fruit, dairy products, meat and fish. This diet may well reduce the amount of bloating and therefore, pain, as it is undigested carbohydrates that ferment in the bowel and cause wind. However, this diet is extremely restricted, tends to be high in saturated fat and could lead to nutritional deficiencies. It should only be undertaken with the help of a qualified dietician.

Dairy-free diet A dairy-free diet means cutting out milk, cheese, yoghurt and all products that contain them. As above, reading the list of ingredients on processed food is essential. Avoid non-fat milk solids, caseinates, whey and lactalbumen, and note that many margarines contain cow's milk derivatives. You may find goat's and sheep's milk products an alternative, but some people are aggravated by them too. Eggs may also cause a problem.

There is now a good range of soya products available, although you may be intolerant of them. Soya milk, unsweetened or sweetened with apple juice, is often organic and may contain added calcium because soya milk is low in this mineral. The taste varies from brand to brand but if you find one you like it's a delicious, healthy (but more expensive) alternative to cow's milk. You can also buy soya yoghurt, soya cheese, soya custard (a good low-fat alternative to ordinary custard) and tofu. The latter is a traditional Japanese product made from soya beans. It is available plain, smoked and marinated and is very versatile. If you are not used to it, however, look for some recipes to give you ideas. (See Appendix 1 for booklist.)

With a dairy-free diet you need to make sure you get all the necessary nutrients from other sources. For example, milk contains vitamin B_{12}, which is hard to get if you don't eat meat, so vegetarians need another source. Cow's milk is also a major source of calcium and this must be obtained from elsewhere.

Candida and IBS

The yeast *Candida albicans* lives in our bowels and as long as our bodies are able to keep it under control it does not create a problem. However, there is a theory that if it gets out of control it causes the symptoms of IBS, particularly diarrhoea, constipation and bloating as well as the more usual vaginal or oral thrush. Both women and men can be affected by candida and you don't have to suffer with thrush to have the problems.

Taking antibiotics, anti-inflammatory drugs such as prednisone and hydrocortisone, the contraceptive pill, oestrogens and steroids encourages candida overgrowth in the large bowel, as does the consumption of refined carbohydrates. It has also been said that people coming off tranquillizers and sleeping pills after long-term use can have candida problems.

Angela says:

'After years of trying virtually everything I was recommended to a naturopath. She told me that from all the symptoms I was showing she was absolutely certain I had candida, and asked if I'd be prepared to go on a very strict elimination diet. I was to eliminate all dairy products, all foods that tend to go mouldy, e.g. mushrooms, and wheat products. This left hardly anything – I was put on short-grain brown rice, all root vegetables and bottled water. This was for four weeks. Then I was able to introduce pulses and herb teas. I was on this diet for seven months, nothing else, and I had vitamin supplements. It was very, very difficult and I lost two stone in weight, but *I didn't have any pain.* My husband was very sceptical and as it was costing a lot of money he was convinced I was being conned; I didn't seem to be getting well because I had a lot of withdrawal symptoms. Then I was asked to give myself enemas once a week to clean the bowel, and all this was removing toxins from my body. It was a very strict and hard regime, but it has paid off for me. I now have less pain from the IBS with much longer periods pain-free, but it hasn't cured it completely.

'I began to reintroduce normal food, but I still don't eat white flour products as I seem to have problems with these. I can have wholemeal flour. I don't eat any red meat at all. All the drugs I had taken over a period of 18 years never solved the problem, in fact most of them made it worse.

'The thing with IBS is that no two people are alike, and I feel that everyone has to try and find their own way of coping with it.'

Chronic candidiasis can affect many parts of the body. The following symptoms, many of which can be long-term, *may* indicate a candida problem:

- Irritable bowel syndrome.
- Fatigue, lethargy, irritability, headaches, migraines.
- Joint pains with or without swelling, muscle pains.
- Nettle rash and hives.
- A history of oral thrush.
- Upper abdominal discomfort or burning.
- Worsening of symptoms after eating refined carbohydrates and heavily yeasted foods.
- Sensitivity to chemicals (petrol fumes, paint, cigarette smoke etc.).
- Craving for refined carbohydrates and/or alcohol.
- Recurrent vaginal thrush/vaginal itching.
- Anal itching.
- Recurrent cystitis.
- Fungal nail or skin infections.
- Iron or zinc deficiency.
- Onset of IBS problems during, or shortly after, pregnancy.
- Sexual partner has candida problems.
- Symptoms precipitated by antibiotics (or a history of repeated or long-term use of antibiotics).

130

- Symptoms worse in low-lying or damp places, near new-mown lawns or raked-up leaves, or on days when the atmosphere is damp (all symptoms of mould allergy).

Much of the list above is rather non-specific, and the same symptoms could be ascribed to many other infections. Consequently, the above symptoms are meant as a guide only.

The role of candida in IBS is controversial and some medical practitioners do not believe it is important. However, it could be that a candida infection may sensitize certain parts of the body, or trigger certain symptoms in an already sensitive part. It could also be that somebody who is very anxious and has a tendency to have IBS also has a rather compromised immune system which allows some candida species to colonize.

So we have the situation where you do not know whether candida is there at all, and, even if it is, you cannot be sure it is a cause of your IBS! All you can do is minimize the chances of candida colonizing your body – in other words, eat for optimal nutrition and minimize stress.

You can try eating garlic – Shirley Trickett recommends eating three crushed cloves a day. [17] They must be taken with yoghurt or milk and washed down with plenty of water, or taken on tomatoes with olive oil. She says that three cloves daily will be 'devastating' for the candida, but you may not feel able to take it raw, especially in view of the smell that will linger on your breath. If you want to try commercial preparations they must contain allicin, which is the anti-fungal substance in the garlic. Sunflower oil, olive oil and food-grade linseed oil (not the sort that artists use, it is poisonous) also have natural anti-yeast and anti-fungal properties. Buy cold-pressed, unrefined oil in small amounts and keep it in the fridge as it can go rancid quickly. These oils are expensive but are really worth getting as they will benefit your immune system too; it is important to do all you can to strengthen your immune system, as only by doing that can you hope for good health. Cut out smoking, alcohol and caffeine, or reduce them if you can't stop all together. (See p. 137 for more on boosting your immune system.)

Some people resort to a course of Nystatin or Mycocidin, two anti-fungal substances. Nystatin must be taken for at least eight weeks to be effective. It is also thought to kill off the candida too quickly; the poisons from the dead cells can make you feel pretty ill. Some researchers feel that Nystatin and other powerful candida agents tend to increase problems rather than curing them.

Candida is fashionable at the moment, and a lot is heard about how an anti-candida diet can help all sorts of disorders. Although there seems to be no medical evidence to suggest that an anti-candida diet is effective in IBS, some people believe it has helped them. Mary says:

'By sheer fluke, I tuned into the end of a TV interview where the miseries of the effects of candida overgrowth were being recounted. Among those mentioned was IBS. I hot-footed it to my nearest bookshop and examined every book mentioning candida. I settled for *Candida Albicans: Could Yeast Be Your Problem?* by Leon Chaitow. There, at last, were many pointers as to why I may have succumbed to IBS, and many hitherto unrelated minor medical problems became understandable – I wasn't a hypochondriac, after all! Hope (again!).

'I decided at this low ebb I had nothing to lose in trying the candida diet – I had long suspected a food link but elimination diets had proved inconclusive. Once I started this diet I realized why – there were so many seemingly innocent products that were riddled with additives, yeasts etc. I couldn't stick rigidly to all the pills and potions recommended as apart from the price being prohibitive many were unavailable, but I cobbled together my own list of vitamin supplements and after three very difficult and hungry months when my weight loss accelerated, I actually began to see an improvement. The discomfort didn't disappear at once. My confidence didn't reassert itself but the diarrhoea ceased and my trips to the loo became far less frequent.

'I cannot pretend that everything is now perfect but, a year on, still adhering strictly to the diet and avoiding cereals which I personally cannot tolerate, I feel so much more in control. After trying so many remedies and feeling so disappointed when each failed, I really would recommend that you try the candida diet. It's not an easy option – it's got to be a serious all-out attempt or it won't work. It takes a long time and it's a very severe diet. I still resent having to miss out on many of life's goodies but when I think of the alternative for me – fear of being embarrassed while in company, in formal meetings, travelling etc. – I'd rather have my life back.'

The anti-candida diet

Just in case you want to try it, the anti-candida diet referred to above is included here.

This diet can be very limiting. It includes cutting out all bread with yeast in it, Marmite and other products containing yeast (such as brewers' yeast and various other supplements, alcohol, cheese (except cottage cheese), mushrooms, food that is not fresh, raisins, sultanas, (in other words anything that is a fungus, is made with mould or may have mould on it); refined carbohydrates – anything with sugar in, all white-flour products (including white bread, biscuits, cakes, white-flour pasta); chocolate; food with vinegar in; citrus fruits or drinks, grapes and grape juice. Limit other fruit to two pieces a day and peel the skin, which contains fungus.

There are different levels of diets, some even more strict, depending on how bad the problem is. Candida overgrowth is often characterized by cravings for the foods that feed the yeast, especially sugar. If you manage to clear the problem up you can slowly go back to your usual diet, but candida will probably come back if you eat a lot of sugar.

It is important that if you are underweight you do not lose more than one or two pounds while on the anti-candida diet. Any problems should be discussed with your doctor. As the anti-candida diet is likely to lead to several nutrient deficiencies it is essential to supplement your diet with vitamins, especially if you are vegetarian. Make sure, of course, that the supplements are yeast-free.

The Hay system

The theory of the Hay System is that because of the different digestive processes involved, starches and sugars should not be eaten at the same meal as proteins and acid fruits. There should be four to four-and-a-half hours between each different meal. However, there is no scientific evidence to support the theory behind this system. Medically speaking, it is not logical – humans have evolved to eat a mixed diet, and it does not seem to make sense to separate starches and sugars from proteins and acid fruits.

Nevertheless, at least the diet recommended is a wholefood one, where vegetables, salads and fruits provide the major part and processed foods are avoided.

Doris Grant and Jean Joice have written a helpful and thorough book about the Hay System which you should consult if you want to give it a go.[18] It provides the theory behind the diet, lists of compatible foods, recipes and menu suggestions.

Dionne says the following about the Hay System diet:

'Because I cook for a growing family and have a full social life I do not follow it strictly, but enough to have cut out most of the pain, the exhaustion of illness, the constipation, heartburn, sleeplessness and build-up of tooth plaque!'

The practicalities of diets

Many supermarkets will provide lists of their products that are free from wheat, gluten, dairy produce, yeast, sugar etc. You can write to the customer relations department of the supermarket chain.

Food allergy associations (see Appendix 2) will give details of suppliers of foods suitable for people who are intolerant of certain substances.

All of these diets are very restrictive and in many cases more expensive because of the need to buy products that are less readily available. There needs to be a move towards providing a better choice of, say, gluten-free products, at a reasonable price and more readily available. Restaurants and cafés also need to be more aware of the needs of those with restrictive diets. If, however, the example of vegetarian products is anything to go by, food that was once considered strange is now on all the supermarket shelves and on all the pub menus, so maybe the future is not too bleak.

The world we live in

Our way of life as part of society, as well as individuals, can have a direct negative effect on our IBS. There was a general feeling among many of the IBS sufferers in our study that there are aspects of the way we live that cause and aggravate IBS, and changes are needed to make the condition easier to deal with.

This is, of course, true of any illness that is affected by stress in any way. Some sentiments are expressed here:

'Less emphasis on the work-till-you-drop attitude.'

'Less pressure and urgency to keep achieving for success's sake. Healthier, greener environment. Less pollution, fewer chemicals in food, household and other products.'

'When I am in safe accommodation with a good financial base, in a job I find enjoyable and stimulating, i.e. when I am materially secure, it will help my IBS.'

'There need to be fewer expectations of the "perfect" mother/ wife/daughter/teacher etc. – we need to accept each other just as we are.'

Rachel describes what caused her IBS:

'At seventeen, unemployed and with no dole, I had no food for months, just ate rarely, what I could get. I smoked and drank a lot.'

Many sufferers feel that more and better public toilets are important for them to be able to cope with their symptoms.

'One becomes aware of the abysmal provision of public toilets and the disgusting habits of The Public! It amuses me when folk return from foreign holidays and complain about the facilities there. I direct them to the one down the road. Supervised lavatories must be provided as the public behave badly in other ones. I am surprised that more fuss is not made in the media about the situation. What a wonderful opportunity for the consumer programmes on TV!' says Tony, an ex-headmaster.

In some places things are going downhill fast. In Sheffield almost all suburban toilets have been closed, as well as several in the town centre. A statement from the City Cleansing Services said that this was due to necessary financial cutbacks and had not been taken lightly – they recognised the concern the decision had caused. The problem is not limited to Sheffield.

Henry says that on his daily drive to work through Manchester he passes at least six or seven closed and boarded-up toilets.

'Suffering from IBS brings home very sharply the quiet scandal of Britain's disappearing public toilets. In tourist areas such as

Cornwall or the Cotswolds I have found provision of toilets generally reasonable, in terms of both number and cleanliness. However, in most of our big towns and cities the opposite is true – toilets are being closed down all over the place for reasons of economy. Within the last couple of years Manchester has closed most of its toilets, apart from those in a handful of shopping centres. My home town of Stockport has just followed suit and announced the closure of two-thirds of the toilets in the borough, and from my travels around the country this seems to be the pattern almost everywhere.

'There must have been a genuine demand for all these toilets when they were built, and with the rise in the number of elderly people, and the obviously large number of IBS sufferers, the overall need, if anything, must have grown. I have read of old people suffering from dehydration, as they are frightened of drinking anything in case they are unable to find a toilet when they are out. Local councillors are inflicting misery on millions of people for paltry savings, in the knowledge that toilets are a subject on which people are too embarrassed to speak out.'

The IBS Network provides a 'Can't Wait' card to all its members. This can be shown in shops and other public places if you need to go to the toilet urgently. It can also be used to skip queues in public toilets without causing bad feeling from others in the queue.

Towards a better life – pushing IBS out of the way

'I'm optimistic my IBS will improve. I believe continuing to identify foods to which I'm sensitive and eliminating them will help. When I feel confident and start making changes in my life I think there could ultimately be improvements in my IBS.'

It is clear that there are no easy answers with IBS. Most of us know that there is no instant cure. Its many symptoms and combinations of symptoms in each of us makes it such a puzzle! How it started, what makes it worse, what part of it is hardest to deal with, what helps – every one of us can tell a different story. No doubt, in time, some people who have been diagnosed as having IBS may be found to be suffering from other conditions. Fifty years ago, what we now call irritable bowel syndrome would have included lactose intolerance, coeliac disease, colitis and bile acid deficiency. If this does happen, some of us may find we don't have IBS but another condition not yet identified and our symptoms may be easily cured. Gastroenterologist Professor Nick Read says, 'The many different presentations of this condition, the non-specific nature of many of the symptoms and the poor and variable response to treatment suggest that irritable bowel syndrome is not more than a convenient clinical category in which to place a large number of patients whose disease mechanisms are poorly understood. Therefore it seems likely that what we call irritable bowel syndrome is not a single disease but consists of many different conditions.'[20]

However, even if this is true, what we have all got in common are:

- Symptoms that are difficult to live with.
- A condition that is poorly understood by doctors and the general public alike.
- A condition that can cause embarrassment and which many people, sufferers and non-sufferers alike, find difficult to talk about.
- A condition that has a poor record of effective treatment.

Meanwhile, the way we live has a significant effect on the health of all of us. Below we look at what steps you can take towards creating optimum health.

Build up your immune system

The immune system is the body's defence against illness. It is made up of an army of special cells ready to go into action at a moment's notice. They attack and destroy anything foreign, from bacteria and viruses to cancers, that invades the body or threatens it from within. If we want good health it is important to know what weakens the immune system and what strengthens it. A well-functioning immune system will help your body to heal itself.

Although science has conquered many serious diseases of the past, there are new threats that our bodies have to face. Chemicals in tap water, pesticides on food and other environmental pollutants weaken our immune systems. This has meant that allergies are on the increase, children especially are more prone to infections, and immunologic diseases, Crohn's disease, multiple sclerosis and rheumatoid arthritis are becoming more common among adolescents.[20]

The key to a healthy immune system is optimal nutrition. Recent research seems to show that we need an adequate intake of essential fatty acids.[21] These are substances that the body cannot manufacture, so they must be obtained from food. It is believed that essential fatty acids (or EFAs) can reduce cholesterol levels in the blood, reduce the risk of heart disease and help sufferers of pre-menstrual syndrome and ME. They are also crucial in the maintenance of the immune system. EFAs are found in food-grade linseed oil, soya, walnut and wheatgerm oil but these must be from a cold climate, fresh, cold-pressed and not hydrogenated. They are also present in salmon, tuna, mackerel, herring and sardines (fresh fish is best as canning causes some loss of essential fatty acids, especially if vegetable oil is used), and dried beans.

Any deficiency of essential minerals and micro-nutrients will depress the immune system, which is why it is important to eat well. Seafood is a rich source of all the minerals, and fresh vegetables will provide the vitamins A and C. These vitamins, as well as zinc and iron, are important boosters of the immune system.

Remember that some drugs depress the immune system; these include steroids, anti-inflammatory drugs and some antibiotics. Stress also depresses the immune system. The health of the immune system is extremely important, and damage to it may make the link with candida and other infections.

Chapter 7

Conclusion and Recommendations

'I am writing to tell you that I feel so much better after coming to the self-help group that I do not need to come any more.'

Having had a glimpse into the lives of other IBS sufferers and looked at the debates around the causes of IBS, you will be wanting to know if there is anything you can do to help alleviate your suffering. It is hard to get on top of a disease or condition if you don't understand it but it is to be hoped that now you have a good understanding of IBS and you can begin to fight back. The following is a brief round-up of everything we have recommended in the previous chapters, along with stories from people who have recovered or almost recovered from IBS which will show you that eliminating IBS is indeed possible.

Medication

While some people respond quite well to drugs, in our experience the relief from symptoms does not last. Drugs may help in the short term, but in the long term we must try to badger the medical profession into finding the causes of IBS, and therefore finding a proper cure. However, until this happens you must decide whether you are going to take medication on a regular basis or for emergencies only, and if so, which. The accent here is on informed choice – why take a drug you know nothing about just because your GP suggests it? Make sure you ask your GP how the drug works and what side-effects are likely. Make sure he or she explains it in simple language, otherwise you will forget what was said as soon as you walk out of the surgery. Appendix IV lists the common drugs used in IBS and explains what they do and the most common side-effects. This should help you in your decision-making.

Melanie found that drugs helped her over some of the bad times:

'My doctor gave me Prothieden, which calmed me and cured my IBS for three months. Although I hate the idea of tranquillizers I think I've come to the conclusion that I prefer them to the discomfort and real suffering of IBS.'

Belle found some of the drugs useful for a time, but does not take them now:

'I had chronic pain and diarrhoea. None of the diarrhoea tablets worked and eventually, after I collapsed on the stairs with exhaustion, the doctor was called. His words as he left my house echoed in my head for ages – "I don't know what to do with you". After a while, we tracked down a private specialist who told me to listen to my body and do what it asks. She placed me on Colofac and Colpermin three times a day, and told me to avoid dairy products as much as possible. I also have a bottle of codeine phosphate which, although it is my lifesaver, doesn't work for everyone. Since I started all this, I am pleased to say that I have made a full recovery now. I am off all tablets.'

Alternative medicine

We cannot recommend any particular alternative therapy which will help IBS sufferers. While some therapies have been said to alleviate the symptoms of IBS, many people still continue to suffer. By all means experiment with different therapies – they are all worth a try – but be careful how you spend your money!

Alternative therapies do not have the same risk of side-effects as does conventional drug treatment and, even if the therapy does not eliminate your symptoms, at the very least you will probably experience an increased feeling of well-being which will help you cope better with your IBS. Ironically, some traditional medical doctors doing research into IBS now feel that a combination of different treatments and a more holistic approach is the way forward for IBS patients.

Although alternative medicine can be very expensive, some practitioners do charge on a sliding scale for people on a low income.

Lifestyle

We know that for some people stress is a trigger factor in IBS, and for all of us stress makes any illness worse. It therefore pays to try to alter your lifestyle so as to minimize stress. Obviously this is very hard to do, especially if you are trying to hold down a job, look after a family, and maybe have financial or other worries as well. There are various books you can buy on relieving stress. A course in stress management may help you, and you may be able to find one at your local adult education institute. Try to include activities in your life which will help you relax – yoga or other relaxing exercise, painting, meditating etc. You need to find interests which will suit you and which you enjoy.

June told us how her IBS has completely disappeared now:

'I am fast approaching my sixtieth year and would not wish to continue to 70 with that complaint, thank you! Now I am definitely not a person who suffers from stress or so I thought. Nevertheless, as luck would have it, my doctor's practice was providing a six-week "Coping with Stress" course at that time, which I promptly joined. I don't know whether it was the effect of being among people who really suffered from stress or the yoga type relaxation exercises we were advised to do, but the IBS disappeared! Now and again, when I am overworked and rushing around more than usual, I do feel a very slight twinge – but that's my warning to slow down, even stop altogether. The memory of that pain is still with me and nothing is worth having that back again.'

Diet

We are asked about diet more than any other topic in our work with IBS sufferers. The short answer is that there is no one diet which will suit all IBS sufferers – you must find out which one suits you best. You should make sure you have a nourishing, well-balanced diet, which is particularly important for people who are often unwell. Variety is the key: do not restrict yourself so much that you allow yourself to be short of nutrients.

Support from others

It is most important to surround yourself with people who are sympathetic and will offer you practical and emotional support when you need it. We advise you to make sure people know of your problems and are sympathetic to you. If they do not take you seriously, they laugh at your symptoms or undermine your confidence, perhaps you should think twice about having them as friends. Make sure you assert yourself and ask for support, both emotional and practical, at times when you need it. Many times people are not sympathetic because they just do not understand your problems and what you are going through. Perhaps they could read this book, or at least look at the following tips on how to deal with the IBS sufferer.

Tips for friends and family
- It may at times be hard to live with a sufferer of IBS. Try to be patient and reassuring. Your partner, relative or friend may suffer with low self-esteem because of her or his IBS. Offer encouragement by telling her or him that you think she or he copes with her or his symptoms well.
- If your partner, friend or relative begins to panic or get a bad pain, speak calmly and reassuringly to her or him. Remind her or him to breathe deeply and, if possible, sit her or him down somewhere quiet where she or he can relax.
- If she or he cannot get to the toilet in time and has an accident, reassure her or him that it doesn't matter and that it happens to many people. Keep the event low-key without denying the distress that she or he may feel. Of course, some people are able to treat an occasional accident as mere inconvenience.
- It helps if you can listen to the sufferer when she or he needs to talk but there may be times, too, when you can help by distracting her or him.
- It is important for her or him to be reassured that she or he is still attractive to you or that you don't find her or him a nuisance or a bore (depending on your relationship!).
- If you live with someone with IBS, be careful not to make the toilet a battleground. Avoid making insensitive

comments about smells, noises, the time she or he takes on the toilet, the number of times she or he has to go back and the inappropriate occasions – such as just as you are about to leave to catch a train, or in the middle of a rush-hour jam on the M25. Believe it or not, this will only make it worse!

Paige is 39 years old, married, with a son and daughter. She describes how her husband speeded her recovery:

'My IBS started about 10 years ago, abroad. I still don't know why, but I had an "accident" when I was out, it was awful, I was so embarrassed. I had abdominal pains and the other symptoms, but there was really nowhere safe to go. After that, I started looking for toilets everywhere – I started having panic attacks on the tube and trains, I didn't know what was happening to me. My doctor thought it was all nerves and sent me to a psychiatrist but he did no good, he didn't understand. Eventually I found it difficult to go out at all, even in the car. Peter was really understanding, though. If we had to come home straight away he never complained. He never made me feel a nuisance or a bother. He was always sympathetic and he went to great pains to reassure me that it wasn't all in my head, I wasn't going mad. He really helped me through. I can't explain it properly; I don't really know how I got better, all I know is that I wouldn't be OK today if it wasn't for him.'

Self-help groups

If there is a self-help group in your area, join it. Even if you only go occasionally you will meet people in the same situation as you, people who understand, and you may pick up some tips for helping your symptoms that you haven't come across before. See Chapter 5 for details of the advantages of self-help groups for people with IBS.

Your GP

Many of our respondents felt their GP was not sympathetic to their needs. If you feel the same way, then *change your doctor*. People often write to us about their problems with their GP, but very few people change to another one. Why is this? If your doctor is not meeting your needs, if you do not feel comfortable with him or her, why stay? Ask your friends and neighbours what they think of their doctors, and ask for a pre-registration interview so that you can find out if the new one is suitable.

Recovery

Through reading this book, you have learnt how sufferers live and cope with their condition. However, the problem with writing a book such as this one is that the people who recover do not generally join IBS groups, or write in with their stories! It is important to realize that many people do recover; one study carried out in 1985 found that after a year 12 per cent of IBS patients were symptom-free, and a further third of them were improved.[1] Only 2 per cent became worse. A follow-up study two to three years later found that half showed substantial improvement. After 6 years, another third of them had no problems. So you can see that people can, and do, get better.

A dual approach

The medical profession as a whole needs to change the way it looks at treating IBS sufferers. As mentioned already, a psychological approach as well as conventional drug treatment has been found to be very valuable for some people. Here is what Dr K. W. Heaton thinks of the dual approach:

'I think the medical profession is slowly progressing in the direction of the dual approach to IBS. However, the great majority of gastroenterologists are completely untrained in psychological treatments. There is also still much uncertainty as to when such treatment should be initiated, how it should be tailored to the individual person and how long it should be continued. A major problem is the severe deficiency of clinical psychologists or even counsellors in the NHS, especially the hospital service.'[2]

Come out!

The best way we can help ourselves in the long term is to increase awareness of IBS among the public, the medical profession, employers, friends and family. We shouldn't have to feel embarrassed about having IBS. The more we talk about it, the more people will understand. When you first have IBS you may think you do not know anyone else who has it, but once you begin to confide in people you will often find they say 'I think I've got that', or 'I had that for two years some time ago', or 'My cousin/sister/mother has that'. It's amazing how many people you will hear about who have IBS. However, some people will have never heard of it, and this is your chance to let them know what IBS is. Increased awareness of IBS can only give good results: it will lead to employers being more sympathetic, and friends and family being more supportive. GPs who at present have little understanding of IBS may begin to see what a devastating effect it can have on people's lives, and how belittled IBS can make us feel. The people who run our councils and are closing down public toilets need educating about IBS, and it is only by all of us raising public awareness that things will improve.

And finally . . .

Finally, here are some points to remember for all-round physical and mental health.

- It is important to remember that in order for the healing process to take place you need to maintain a positive attitude. Easier said than done, you cry! And don't we know it. However, the more you can do yourself to improve your health, the better. Taking responsibility is part of taking control, and those of us with IBS soon realize that we can't rely on the medical profession. It's up to us. Make sure you are open to experiencing an improvement in your symptoms. In other words, don't assume, at any time, that you will feel bad before you actually do.
- If you've found it difficult to talk about your IBS, consider

making contact with other sufferers through the IBS Network, as penpals, phone pals, or meeting them personally. It is important to have someone to turn to.

- All treatment for IBS should take into account the whole person – mind and body.
- Remember that stress can make all illnesses worse, not just IBS.
- Avoid resorting to laxatives. If they are used regularly the bowel becomes lazy and will eventually be unable to function without them.
- Avoid antibiotics that aren't necessary. In fact, only take medical drugs if you really have to. This includes prescription and over-the-counter drugs. Some can make the symptoms of IBS worse in the long term.
- Smoking can cause a number of problems for anyone with abdominal trouble. It intensifies gas and stimulates intestinal activity. In addition, the nicotine reduces the blood flow to the digestive system, which can aggravate abdominal pain and spasms.
- Recreational or street drugs have a negative effect on your health.
- Take regular physical exercise. Try to do something that you enjoy! You will no doubt experience an increased sense of well-being that will help you cope with your life in general, as well as IBS. Aim for three to four episodes of moderately strenuous exercise for 40 to 60 minutes each week. If this is new to you, work up to it gradually. If you can't manage that, any amount of regular exercise is worthwhile. And here's something to think about – Dr Vernon Coleman, in his book *Bodypower*, says, 'One of the ironies of modern living is that many people who don't take enough exercise, and who use gadgets daily to help avoid exercise, spend a lot of money on rowing machines, exercise bicycles and other devices designed to help them get some exercise!'[3]
- Mental exercise is also important and there is no doubt that mental and physical health are bound up together. Stimulate your mind with creativity, hobbies, reading. Again, do things you enjoy.

- Both mental and physical exercise can help to take your mind off your symptoms. This is particularly important to those of us who know there is a direct connection between thinking about our IBS and suddenly wanting to dash to the toilet!
- Concentrate on the areas of your life where you feel in control. You may not be able to go to football matches with your friends but you can build the model train set you always wanted. You may not be able to be relied upon to go on your child's school coach trip but you can be counted on for a cuddle and a bedtime story. Carry this through to all areas of your life – at work, at home, in your relationships.
- Remember that life can be enjoyed and that it is possible to experience pleasure even if you are unwell. When you feel really low, concentrate on the areas of your life which make you feel good and know that you are helping your body to heal.

Although you cannot cure yourself of all of your symptoms, we hope that the information in this book will help you overcome the anxiety, distress and isolation you may have felt because of your condition. You *can* overcome the disabling physical and psychological effects of IBS, even while your symptoms remain. Be optimistic – research is being carried out today which may one day make life easier for everyone with IBS. Meanwhile, we must help ourselves.

Appendix I

Further Reading

Irritable bowel syndrome

Nicol, R., *Coping Successfully with your Irritable Bowel*, Sheldon Press, London, 1989.

Nicol, R., *The Irritable Bowel Diet Book*, Sheldon Press, London, 1990.

Nicol, R., *The Irritable Bowel Stress Book*, Sheldon Press, London, 1991.

Thompson, W. Grant, *Gut Reactions: Understanding Symptoms of the Digestive Tract*, Plenum Press; London, 1989.

Trickett, S., *Irritable Bowel and Diverticulosis: A Self-Help Plan*, Thorsons, London, 1990.

Watts, G. *The Irritable Bowel Syndrome: A Practical Guide*, Cedar Press, London, 1990.

Nutrition

Davies, S. and Stewart, A., *Nutritional Medicine*, Pan, London, 1987.

Galland, L., *Allergy Prevention for Kids*, Bloomsbury, London, 1989.

Brostoff, J. and Gamlin, L., *The Complete Guide to Food Allergy and Intolerance*, Bloomsbury, London, 1989.

Grant, D. and Joice, J., *Food Combining for Health*, Thorsons, London, 1984.

Special interest

Jacobs, G., *Candida Albicans: Yeast and your Health*, Optima, London, 1990.

Useful Addresses

Bowel disorders

British Digestive Foundation, 3 St Andrews Place, Regent's Park, London NW1 4LB.

British Society of Gastroenterology, 3 St Andrews Place, Regent's Park, London NW1 4LB.

Continence Foundation, 380–4 Harrow Rd, London W9 2HU. SAE and donation towards costs appreciated.

Crohns Disease and Colitis Association of South Australia, 32 Reid Avenue, Tranmere 5073, South Australia. Contact secretary Maggie Noble for information about IBS.

International Foundation for Bowel Dysfunction, PO Box 17864, Milwaukee, Wisconsin 53217, USA. Produces a newsletter, *Participate*, for people affected by bowel dysfunction or incontinence.

National Incontinence Helpline. 091–213 0050 (Mon–Fri 2–7pm). A confidential service for people whose lives are affected by incontinence. The telephone line is staffed by health professionals.

Pain

Campain, 26 Weston Rise, Caister, Norfolk NR30 5AT. (Charity created by doctors and health professionals aiming to change attitudes towards pain and improve its relief.)

Self-Help In Pain (SHIP), 33 Kingsdown Park, Whitstable, Kent CT5 2DT. Phone helpline: 0227 264677.

Unwind, 'Melrose', 3 Alderlea Close, Gilesgate, Durham DH1 1DS. (For and by sufferers of pain in its various forms: physical, emotional and mental. A self-help group that publishes a newsletter three times a year.)

Allergy and food intolerance

Action Against Allergy, 24/26 High Street, Hampton Hill, Middx TW12 1PD. A self-help group that publishes a newsletter and provides information; send a large SAE.

National Society for Research into Allergy, PO Box 45, Hinkley, Leicestershire, LE10 1JY. Provides information on the management of allergies.

Producers and suppliers of dairy-free, gluten-free and other products

Berrydales, Berrydale House, 5 Lawn Rd, London NW3 2XS. Tel: 071–722 2866. Producers of dairy, gluten- and egg-free products, including dairy-free ices.

The Candida Shop, Natural Ways, Arfryn, Caergeiliog, Anglesey, Gwynedd LL65 3NL. Sells various products and advises on candida problems. Fee for a consultation by post.

Ener-G, General Designs Ltd, PO Box 38E, Worcester Park, Surrey KT4 7LX. (Produces gluten-free food.)

Food Watch International Ltd, Pollards Yard, Wood Street, Taunton, Somerset, TA1 1UP. Tel:0823 325023. Manufacturers and importers of specialist dietary foods such as gluten-free, egg-free, grain-free, vegan, yeast-free, low-fat and low-sodium. None of their foods contain wheat, cow's milk or any of its derivatives. They can give details of nearest suppliers.

Green Farm Natural Health Products, Burwash Common, E. Sussex TN19 7LX. (Provides a mail order service for a variety of products, including colon-cleansing herbs.)

Nutricia Dietary Products Ltd, 494–496 Honeypot Lane, Stanmore, Middx HA7 1JH. Gluten-free products.

Sun Yums, 52 Kenilworth Rd, Fleet, Hants GU13 9AZ. Gluten-free products.

Trufree Foods, Larkhall Natural Health, 225 Putney Bridge Rd, London SW15 2PY. Tel: 081-874 1130. Gluten-free products, including bread and cake mixes, and a free handbook for coeliacs and gluten-free/wheat-free dieters, *Getting Safely Started*.

Ultrapharm Ltd, PO Box 18, Henley-on-Thames, Oxfordshire RG9 2AW. Gluten-free products.

Appendix II

Anxiety

First Steps To Freedom, 22 Randall Road, Kenilworth, Warwickshire, CV8 1JY. A charity which aims to help phobics, anxiety sufferers, those who suffer from obsessive and compulsive disorders and their carers, and those who wish to come off tranquillizers. Telephone helplines:

Warwickshire: 0926 351603
Derbyshire: 0332 760982
Shropshire: 0952 590545

Holistic medicine

British Acupuncture Association & Register, 34 Alderney Street, London SW1V 4EU. Will provide a list of registered practitioners.

British Holistic Medical Association, 179 Gloucester Place, London NW1 6DX.

British Homeopathic Association, 27A Devonshire St, London W1. Will provide a list of registered practitioners as well as information on homeopathy. Enclose an SAE.

British Hypnotherapy Association, 1 Wythburn Place, London W1. Hypnotherapy for emotional problems, relationship difficulties, neurotic behaviour patterns, sex problems, phobias etc. Can provide a list of trained, registered hypnotherapists in your area, plus information pamphlet if you send details about your problem and enclose £2. Also provides various publications on hypnotherapy: send SAE for list.

British Society of Medical and Dental Hypnosis, 42 Links Rd, Ashtead, Surrey KT21 2HJ.

General Council and Register of Consultant Herbalists, Marlborough House, Swanpool, Falmouth, Cornwall TR11 4HW.

Institute for Complementary Medicine, PO Box 194, London SE16 1QZ. (Holds the British Register of Complementary Practitioners. Enclose an SAE.)

National Institute of Medical Herbalists, 41 Hatherley Rd, Winchester SO22 6SR

International Federation of Aromatherapists, Department of Continuing Education, The Royal Masonic Hospital, Ravenscourt Park, London W6 0TN. Tel: 081-846 8066.

Mrs E. E. Taylor, BSc (Hons) offers private sessions of Specialist (gut-directed) hypnotherapy for IBS. Telephone: 0706 312041.

Food

Foresight (The Association for Promotion of Preconceptual Care),
Mrs Peter Barnes, 28 The Paddock, Godalming, Surrey, GU7 1XD.
(Primarily an organization to promote good health of parents prior
to conception, but publishes a booklet, *Findout*, listing all additives
and E numbers and their known dangers.

National Centre for Organic Gardening, Ryton-on-Dunsmore, Coventry,
CV8 3LG. (Information on local wholefood and organic suppliers.)

While every care has been taken in compiling this list, we cannot accept
responsibility for any error or mis-statement contained therein.

Appendix III

The IBS Network

The IBS Network was founded in 1991 by Susan Backhouse and Christine Dancey in order to help alleviate the distress, suffering and isolation associated with irritable bowel syndrome. Until then there had been no self-help organization for sufferers of the condition, and we have been unable to find a similar one in any other country.

Members receive the quarterly newsletter *Gut Reaction*, which includes information about the growing network of local IBS self-help groups. There are also 'befriending' and penpal schemes for members.

For more information, please send an SAE to IBS Network, c/o The Wells Park Health Project, 1a Wells Park Rd, London, SE26 6JE.

Glossary of Drug Treatments

Alimix	Cisapride. Facilitates or restores gastric motility. Do not take if pregnant, or with anti-cholinergic drugs. Side effects can include abdominal cramps, rumbling noises in digestive system and diarrhoea.
Amitryptyaline	Anti-depressant. Has a sedative effect.
Bolvidion	For depression. Not for nursing mothers. May cause drowsiness.
Buscopan	An anti-cholinergic anti-spasmodic. Can cause blurred vision, dry mouth.
Carbellon	Anti-cholinergic/antacid/anti-flatulant. Contains charcoal, peppermint oil.
Codeine Phosphate	Used as an analgesic to relieve pain. Codeine is a weak narcotic – low potential for addiction.
Colofac	Meteverine hydrochlor. Anti-spasmodic.
Colpermin	Anti-spasmodic. Helps to relieve discomfort due to excessive wind by encouraging eructation (belching). Contains peppermint oil. Can be bought over the counter.
Colven	Anti-spasmodic and bulking agent, for IBS.

Diconal

Opiate. Used for moderate to severe pain. Should not be used when pregnant. Do not use with alcohol. Side effects: drowsiness, dry mouth. Addictive.

Dolmatil

Sulpiride. Sedative to treat schizophrenia. Side effects: muscle spasms, dry mouth, urine retention, weight gain, drowsiness, menstrual changes, jaundice. Not to be used with a variety of other drugs including alcohol, painkillers, tranquillizers and anti-depressants.

Dothiepin (Prothiaden)

Anti-depressant. Side effects: dry mouth, constipation, blurred vision, drowsiness, sleeplessness, dizziness, weight change, loss of libido (sex drive).

Dulcolax

Tablets or suppositories for treatment of constipation or to empty the bowel prior to medical examination.

Duphalac (Lactulose)

Osmotic laxative to treat constipation. Take with plenty of water.

Fybogel

Bulking agent to counteract constipation.

Imipramine (Tofranil)

Anti-depressant. Side effects: as for Dothiepin.

Imodium

Loperamide. Anti-diarrhoeal agent. An opiate. Slows down the passage of intestinal contents so that more water is reabsorbed into the body.

Isogel

Bulking agent for constipation or diarrhoea.

Kolanticion

For gastrointestinal spasms, flatulence, hyperacidity. Can cause constipation, dry mouth.

Lactulose (See Duplac)

Lentizol (Amitriptyline hydrochloride) — For depression. Side effects: as for Dothiepin.

Librium — Tranquillizer – treats anxiety. Causes drowsiness. Side effects: confusion, unsteadiness, changes in vision and sex drive, retention of urine. Addictive. Not to be used long-term, and withdrawal should be gradual.

Loperamide — See Imodium.

Merbentyl — Anti-cholinergic anti-spasmodic for bowel and stomach spasm. Can cause blurred vision, dry mouth.

Mogadon — Sleeping tablet. Sedation may carry through to next day. Side effects: confusion, unsteadiness, rash, changes in vision and sex drive, retention of urine. Not to be used long-term, withdraw gradually. Not to be used with alcohol, other tranquillizers or anti-convulsants.

Motival (Fluphenazine hydrochlor) — Phenothiazine. For anxiety/depression. Side effects: as for Dothiepin.

Normacol — Bulking agent.

Regulan — Bulking agent to relieve constipation due to lack of dietary fibre.

Senokot — Stimulant to treat constipation. Increases colonic mobility. May cause colicky pain in the long term. Should only be used on specific occasions.

Spasmonal — Anti-spasmodic. Can cause dry mouth, blurred vision, confusion.

Sulpiride — See Dolmatil.

Trytizol (Amitriptyline hydrochloride) — Anti-depressant. Side effects: as for Dothiepin.

Valium   Tranquillizer – treats anxiety.
                              Causes drowsiness. Side effects:
                              reduced reactions. Not to be used
                              long-term and withdrawal should be
                              gradual.

References

Preface

1. Almy, T.P. and Rothstein, R.I., IBS: classification and pathogenesis, *Annual Review of Medicine*, 1987, 38, 257–65.
2. Whitehead, W.E., Winget, C., Fedoravicius, A.S., Wooley, S. and Blackwell, B., Learned illness behaviour in patients with IBS and peptic ulcer, *Digestive Diseases and Sciences*, 1982, 27, 202–8.
3. Switz, D.M., What the gastroenterologist does all day. A survey of a state society's practice, *Gastroenterology*, 1977, 70, 1048–50.
4. Walker, E.A., Roy-Byrne, P.P. and Katon, W.J., IBS and psychiatric illness, *American Journal of Psychiatry*, 1990, 147, 5, 565–72.

Chapter 1

1. Thompson, W. Grant, *Gut Reactions: Understanding Symptoms of the Digestive Tract*, Plenum Press, London, 1989.
2. Almy, T.P. and Rothstein, R.I., IBS: classification and pathogenesis, *Annual Review of Medicine*, 1987, 38, 257–65.
3. Thompson, W.G. and Heaton, K.W., Functional bowel disorders in apparently healthy people, *Gastroenterology*, 1980, 79, 283–8.
4. *Ibid.*
5. Manning, A.P., Thompson, W.G., Heaton, K.W., Moris, A.F., Towards a positive diagnosis of the irritable bowel, *British Medical Journal*, 1978, 2, 653–4.
6. Endometriosis Association, Newsletter, 1988, 9, 1, USA.

References

7. Thompson, W. Grant, *Gut Reactions: Understanding Symptoms of the Digestive Tract*, Plenum Press, London, 1989.

8. Wingate, D.L., The brain-gut link, *Viewpoints on digestive diseases*, 1985, 17, 5, 17–20.

9. McCloy, R. and McCloy, E., *The IBS: Clinical Perspectives*, Meditext Ltd, London, 1988.

10. Soffer, E.E., Scalabrini, P., Pope II, C.E. and Wingate, D.L., Effect of stress on oesophageal motor function in normal subjects and in patients with the irritable bowel syndrome, *Gut*, 1986, 29, 11, 1591–4.

11. Kellow, J.E., Gill, R.C. and Wingate, D.L., Prolonged ambulant recordings of small bowel motility demonstrate abnormalities in the irritable bowel syndrome, *Gastroenterology*, 1990, 98, 1208–18.

12. Read, N.W., IBS: One disease or several? The identification of pathophysiological subsets, *Current Approaches towards Confident Management of Irritable Bowel Syndrome*, Duphar Medical Relations, Southampton, 1991.

13. Apley, J., *The Child with Recurrent Abdominal Pains* (2nd ed), Blackwell Scientific, Oxford, 1975.

14. Prior, A., Stanley, K., Smith, A.R.B. and Read, N.W., The relationship between hysterectomy and the irritable bowel: a prospective study, *Gut*, 1992, 33, 814–17.

15. Taylor, T., Smith, A.N. and Fulton, P.M., Effect of hysterectomy on bowel function, *British Medical Journal*, 1989, 299, 300–1.

16. Read, N.W., Personal communication, 1992.

17. Dyson, R., *Gut Reaction 7*, The IBS Network, Sheffield, 1992.

18. Latimer, P., Psychophysiologic disorders: a critical appraisal of concept and theory illustrated with reference to the irritable bowel syndrome (IBS), *Psychological Medicine*, 1979, 9, 1, 71–80.

19. Mitchell, M.C. and Drossman, D.A., The IBS: Understanding and treating a biopsychosocial illness disorder, *Annals of Behavioral Medicine*, 1987, 9, 3, 13–18.

Chapter 2

1. Heaton, K.W., O'Donnell, L., Braddon, F., Mountford, R., Hughes, A, and Cripps, P.J., Irritable bowel syndrome in a British urban community: consulters and non-consulters, *Gastroenterology*, 1992, 102, 1962–7.

2. *Ibid*.
3. Thompson, W. Grant., *Gut Reactions: Understanding Symptoms of the Digestive Tract*, Plenum Press, London, 1989.
4. McCloy, R. and McCloy, E., *The IBS: Clinical Perspectives*, Meditext Ltd, London, 1988.
5. *Ibid*.
6. Mallinson, C., Personal communication, 1991.

Chapter 3

1. McCloy, R. and McCloy, E., *The IBS: Clinical Perspectives*, Meditext Ltd, London, 1988.
2. Kellow, J.E., Gill, R.C. and Wingate, D.L., Prolonged ambulant recordings of small bowel motility demonstrate abnormalities in the irritable bowel syndrome, *Gastroenterology*, 1990, 98, 1208–18.
3. Ford, M.J., Invited review: the irritable bowel syndrome, *Journal of Psychosomatic research*, 1986, 30, 4, 399–410.
4. Thompson, W. Grant, *Gut Reactions: Understanding Symptoms of the Digestive Tract*, Plenum Press, London 1989.
5. Trickett, S., *IBS and Diverticulosis: A Self-help Plan*, Thorsons, London, 1990.
6. Read, N., Personal communication, 1993.
7. Eating Disorders Association, *Prevent Laxative Abuse Now* (PLAN) Information Pack, 1992.
8. Ritchie, J.A. and Truelove, S.C. Comparison of various treatments for IBS, *British Medical Journal*, 1980, 281, 1317–19.
9. Blanchard, E.B., Schwartz, S.P. and Radnitz, C.L., Psychological assessment and treatment of irritable bowel syndrome, *Behavior Modification*, 1987, 11, 3, 348–72.
10. Guthrie, E., Creed, F., Dawson, D. and Tomenson, B., A controlled trial of psychological treatment for the irritable bowel syndrome, *Gastroenterology*, 1991, 100, 450–7.
11. Whorwhell, P.J., A pathophysiological approach to the management of irritable bowel syndrome, *Horizons in Medicine III*, ed. Summerfield, J.A. and Seymour, C. Royal College of Physicians, 1991.
12. *Ibid*.
13. Mallinson, C., Personal communication, 1991.
14. Whorwhell, P.J., A pathophysiological approach to the management of irritable bowel syndrome, *Horizons in Medicine III*,

ed. Summerfield, J.A. and Seymour, C. Royal College of Physicians, 1991.

15. Cotterell, J.C., Lee, A.J., and Hunter, J.O., Double-blind cross-over trial of evening primrose oil in women with menstrually-related irritable bowel syndrome, *Pathophysiology and Roles in Clinical Medicine*, 1990, 31, 421–6.

16. McCloy, R. and McCloy, E., *The IBS: Clinical Perspectives*, Meditext Ltd, London, 1988.

17. Mallinson, C., Personal communication, 1991.

18. Read, N.W., Personal communication, 1992.

19. Broome, A. and Jellicoe, H., *Living with your Pain: A Self-help Guide to Managing Pain*, Methuen & Co, London, 1987.

20. Trickett, S., *IBS and Diverticulosis: A Self-help Plan*, Thorsons, London, 1990.

Chapter 4

1. Kumar, D., Pfeffer, J. and Wingate, D.L., Role of psychological factors in the irritable bowel syndrome, *Digestion*, 1990, 45, 80–7.

2. Corney, R.H. and Stanton, R., Physical symptom severity, psychological and social dysfunction in a series of outpatients with IBS, *Journal of Psychosomatic Research*, 1990, 34, 5, 483–91.

Chapter 5

1. Corney, R.H. and Stanton, R., Physical symptom severity, psychological and social dysfunction in a series of outpatients with IBS, *Journal of Psychosomatic Research*, 1990, 34, 5, 483–91.

2. Cook, I.J., Van Eeden, A. and Collins, S.M., Patients with IBS have greater pain tolerance than normal subjects, *Gastroenterology*, 1987, 93, 4, 727–33.

3. Brice, Judith, M.D., Psychological aspects of living with a chronic intestinal illness, *Intestinal Fortitude*, 1990–1, Winter, USA.

4. Ganster, D.C. and Victor, B., The impact of social support on mental and physical health. Special Issue: stress and health, *British Journal of Medical Psychology*, 1988, 61, 1, 17–36.

5. Revenson, T.A., Schiaffino, K.M., Majerovitz, S.D., and Gibofsky, A., Social support as a double-edged sword: the relation of positive

and problematic support to depression among rheumatoid arthritis patients, *Social science and medicine*, 1991, 33, 7, 807–13.

Chapter 6

1. Whitehead, W.E. and Bosmajian, L.S., Behavioral medical approaches to gastrointestinal disorders, *Journal of Consulting & Clinical Psychology*, 1982, 50, 6, 972–83.
2. *Ibid.*
3. Drossman, D.A., Sandler, R.S., McKee, D.C. et al., Bowel patterns among subjects not seeking health care, *Gastroenterology*, 1982, 38, 529–34.
4. Kumar, D., Pfeffer, J. and Wingate, D.L., Role of psychological factors in the irritable bowel syndrome *Digestion*, 1990, 45, 80–87
5. Heaton, K.W., Creed, F. and Goeting, N.L.M. (eds), *Current Approaches towards confident Management of Irritable Bowel Syndrome*, Duphar Medical Relations, Southampston, 1991.
6. Holmes, T.H. and Rahe, R.H., The social readjustment ratings scale, *Journal of Psychosomatic Research*, 1967, 11, 213–18.
7. Lydiard, R.B., Loraia, M.T., Howell, E.F. and Ballenger, J.C. can panic disorder present as irritable bowel syndrome, *Journal of Clinical Psychiatry*, 1986, 47, 9, 470–3.
8. Coleman, V., *Bodypower*, Thames & Hudson, London 1983.
9. Heaton, K.W., Creed, F. and Goeting, N.L.M. (eds), *Current Approaches towards Confident Management of Irritable Bowel Syndrome* Duphar Medical Relations Southampton, 1991.
10. Bennett, P. and Wilkinson, S., A comparison of psychological and medical treatment of the irritable bowel syndrome, *British Journal of Clinical Psychology*, 1985, 24, 215–16.
11. Guthrie, E. *Current Approaches Towards Confident Management of Irritable Bowel Syndrome*, Duphar Medical Relations, Southampton, 1991.
12. The Association for Promotion of Preconceptual care, *Findout*, Foresight, Surrey, 1986.
13. Galland, L., *Allergy Prevention for Kids*, Bloomsbury, London 1988
14. *Ibid.*
15. Cann, P., Read, N.W. and Holdsworth, C.D., What is the benefit of coarse wheat bran in patients with irritable bowel syndrome? *Gut*, 1984, 25, 168–73.

16. McCloy, R. and McCloy, E., *The IBS: Clinical Perspectives*, Meditext Ltd, London, 1988.
17. Trickett, S., *IBS and Diverticulosis: A Self-help Plan* Thorsons, London, 1990.
18. Grant, D & Joice, J., *Food Combining For Health*, Thorsons, London, 1984.
19. Read, N., Personal correspondence, 1992.
20. Read, N., IBS: One disease or several? The identification of pathophysiological sub sets, *Current Approaches towards Confident Management of Irritable Bowel Syndrome*, Heaton, K.W., Creed, F. and Goeting, N.L.M. (eds), Duphar Medical Relations, Southampton, 1991.
21. Galland, L., *Allergy prevention for kids*, Bloomsbury, London, 1988.
22. *Ibid.*

Chapter 7

1. Langeluddecke, P.L., Psychological aspects of irritable bowel syndrome, *Australian and New Zealand Journal of Psychiatry* 1985, 19, 3, 218–26.
2. Read, N., Personal communication, 1992.
3. Coleman, V., *Bodypower*, Thames & Hudson, London, 1983.